GOD'S WILL BE DONE
VOLUME II

MORAL HEALER'S HANDBOOK:
THE PSYCHOLOGY OF SPIRITUAL CHIVALRY

LALEH BAKHTIAR

FOREWORD BY

SEYYED HOSSEIN NASR

THE INSTITUTE OF TRADITIONAL
PSYCHOETHICS AND GUIDANCE

Library of Congress Cataloging in Publication Data

Bakhtiar, Laleh
    Moral Healer's Handbook: The Psychology of
    Spiritual Chivalry. Volume 2: God's Will Be Done

    Includes bibliographical references.
    1. Psychology, Religious. 2. Consciousness. 3. Ethics. 4.
Counseling. I. Bakhtiar, Laleh. II. Title.
BL53.U45   200'.1975.16302
ISBN: 1871031397 (pbk)

Book Designer
Liaquat Ali

Published by:
The Institute of Traditional Psychoethics and Guidance

Distributed by:
KAZI Publications, Inc.
3023 W. Belmont Ave Chicago IL 60618
Tel: 312-267-7001 FAX: 312-267-7002

CONTENTS

*"And as for those who struggle (perform the **Jihād**) in Our Cause, surely We guide them in Our Ways"* **(29:69).**

To my spiritual warrior who has been so guided.

FOREWORD

The contemporary religious scene is characterized not only by the survival and in some cases revival of the traditions which have been the millennial gardens of wisdom, but also new so-called religious and spiritual currents usually associated with a "teacher" who declares his independence of any sacred tradition and presents himself ultimately as a new "prophet." Of dubious pedigree and origin, many such movements claim at the same time to have received, refined and made available some of the esoteric practices and doctrines of the religious traditions, practices and doctrines which they then present independently of the framework within which they possess full meaning. Some of these techniques and practices still possess at least some efficacy even outside of the sacred cadre where they naturally belong, while others are most dangerous and only contribute to the psychological imbalance and spiritual confusion which characterizes today's world.

One such technique is meditation upon and the study of the Enneagram which is now used widely as help for psychological healing and even "spiritual advancement." Made popular by some of the self-appointed gurus and "teacher" of the earlier part of this century and some who are still active today, it has also spread among Christians especially Catholics, millions of whom use it regularly but few have bothered to delve into the traditional origin of the Enneagram and the significant role that it has played in the traditional sacred universe.

It is the virtue of this book to have dealt for the first time with this theme and to have revealed the origin of the Enneagram as used in spiritual practice and moral healing in the Islamic tradition. The author deals in detail with the spiritual significance of the Saturn-Jupiter cycle in Islamic symbolic astrology as developed by the Sufis, especially Ibn 'Arabī, and the relation of this cycle to the Enneagram. She also brings other important evidence to bear upon the Islamic origin of the Enneagram as used in spiritual practice, making use of not only Sufi texts but also works of philosophical ethics such as those of Naṣir al-Din Tūsī.

The greatest contribution of the book, however, is to situate the use of the Enneagram within the context of the Islamic tradition of spiritual chivalry. Known as *futuwwah* (in Arabic) or *javanmardī* (in Persian), spiritual chivalry is of the utmost significance for the understanding of the spiritual life of Islam. Associated originally in the Quran with the

Prophet Abraham, it is embodied in the Islamic tradition itself with 'Alī ibn Abī Tālib, who plays such a pivotal role, as heir to the esoteric teachings of the Prophet of Islam in not only the Sufi orders but also the guilds and orders of knightly chivalry. Spiritual chivalry means a continuous spiritual warfare by means of which the soul of the human being becomes imbued with the virtues that heal the wounds of the fallen soul and prepare it for the encounter with God.

The author re-integrates the meaning and practical use of the Enneagram into the traditional Islamic framework from which it issued. She develops fully the doctrine of the correspondence between the macrocosm and the microcosm which, in fact, makes possible the use of such a symbol and is the basis for its efficacy within a living spiritual tradition. In doing so, not only does she provide knowledge concerning the historical origin of the Enneagram as an instrument for moral and psychological healing and spiritual development, she also emphasizes in this connection, the role of moral and spiritual virtues so characteristic of spiritual chivalry, thereby refuting the claim to the possibility of the amoral use of this and other spiritual techniques and methods employed in so many non-traditional circles today.

Dr. Bakhtiar is to be congratulated in clarifying an aspect of Islamic spirituality as imbedded in spiritual chivalry and many basic metaphysical and cosmological doctrines of Islamic esotericism, as well as in bringing out the full meaning and spiritual import of the Enneagram. Her work, therefore, possesses not only a scholarly significance but also a practical one for those who are making practical use of the Enneagram and who are in quest of means to achieve moral and psychological healing. The book also conveys the very significant message that traditional techniques, doctrines and symbols, while always possessing an innate value which issues from their very nature grounded in the Truth, reveal their full meaning and efficacy only within a living spiritual universe although they can also be transmitted from one such universe to another.

We hope that the present book reaches all those who are interested seriously in the meaning of the Enneagram and who are looking for means of healing the soul outside of the ordinary channels in the modern world which has caused so many scars upon the souls of so many people at the same time that it is so bereft of the means of healing these scars because it has forgotten the basic distinction between the Spirit and the soul and the crucial fact that only the Spirit has the ability to heal the wounds of the soul in a world separated from its Divine Origin.

Seyyed Hossein Nasr
Washington, D. C., May, 1994

PREFACE

To speak of tradition is to speak of the timeless, religion in its most universal sense. The universal sense of religion incorporates both the Law and the Way. While the Law is the outer dimension, the Way is the inner. This work is encompassed by the inner dimension or the Way, never forgetting that the door to the Way is through the Law. The Law and the Way provide the rules for executing the trust of nature given to the human being, the trustee being the morally healed spiritual warrior.

Spiritual chivalry (*futuwwah*) grew out of traditional societies. It is the model for the humanity that is "the middle way," the model for the humanity that shall inherit the earth. It means "moral goodness" and is based in the psychology of ethics or as the author terms it, "psychoethics."

The stages the spiritual warrior moves through are moral goodness (*murūwwah*), spiritual chivalry (*futuwwah*) and sanctity or being a friend of God (*walāyah*). As the concept unfolds for the reader, it becomes more and more familiar to people from the Judeo-Christian-Islamic or monotheistic tradition and yet it is not unknown to the Japanese samurai or the followers of Confucius and Lao Tse.

Traditional models are plentiful for the spiritual warrior beginning with Prophet Abraham, who is referred to in the Quran as a spiritual warrior when he destroys the idols. Other models include the foster-mother of Moses, Asiyah, and the Virgin Mary, Prophet Jesus, the Seven Sleepers or the Companions of the Cave, the Messenger Muhammad and his wife Khadijah. It is essentially anyone who manifests the moral reasonableness of a person cultured by monotheism (*hilm*) as opposed to someone who manifests what is known as ignorance (*jahl*) of the Real workings of the universe.

ix

Spiritual chivalry as the model for moral healing is the basis for what is known in the West as the Enneagram and what the Sufis call "the Presence of God" (*wajh Allāh*). It is a model which arises out of a traditional society where correspondences are sought between the microcosm and the macrocosm as so many Signs of God's Presence or symbols interpreted through spiritual hermeneutics (*ta'wil*).

While the Sign of the Presence of God symbolizes the human "self" on the microcosmic plane, its macrocosmic correspondence in spiritual astrology is presented here for the first time in the West because according to spiritual hermeneutics, all sciences are of Divine origin and have their base in the sciences of numbers, geometry and letters. This is true of the science of psychoethics as well as spiritual alchemy and its macrocosmic counterpart, spiritual astrology, which are discussed in their relationship to spiritual chivalry.

In spite of the presence of many models, the reason for the increase of emphasis upon this model in certain periods of history and a decline in others is because the model had been connected to psychoethics in oral tradition. That is, it has traditionally depended upon the strength or weaknesses of the spiritual masters and the encouragement or lack of encouragement of the rulers.

Once the Sign of "the Presence of God" became readily available in the West in the early 20th century under the name of the Enneagram, studies in recent times began to flourish on it as a possible typology. However, these studies have lost touch with the origins of the model of spiritual chivalry at the stage of attaining moral goodness (*murūwwah*) and its basis in psychoethics. Therefore, it has moved in a direction of interpretation of what it might mean but not what it has meant in the Sufi tradition.

With this work as an extension of *God's Will Be Done: Traditional Psychoethics and Personality Paradigm*, awareness of the self-help method of moral healing through spiritual struggle towards attaining spiritual chivalry is clearly delineated and its base in traditional psychoethics. There are many practices developed within the discipline of spiritual chivalry but the major one upon which the Sign of "the Presence of God" rests is that of the greater struggle (*jihād al-akbar*). This is the most important of the practices for our purposes. The process is through exposing one's own state of ignorance (*jahl*) of Reality and replacing this state with a state of the moral reasonableness of a religiously cultured monotheist (*ḥilm*). It begins and ends each day through self-examination by knowing self and one's Lord until the next day when the cycle begins again. It is this practice of "remembrance" to which the Sign of the Presence of God relates as a self-help method of moral healing through continuous self-examination."

*

My thanks to my children Mani, Davar, Susan, Karim, Shervin and Farroukh for their support along with my brother, Jamshid and sister Shireen Bakhtiar (whose pen name is White Cloud). I wish to offer a special prayer for my two beloved grandchildren, Saied and Samira, who I pray will someday manifest the model of spiritual chivalry like the spiritual warrior who inspired this work. I also wish to express my appreciation to my teachers: Javad Nurbakhsh, Seyyed Hossein Nasr and Jamshid Bakhtiar. Arabic translations were done with the help of Muhammad al-Akili and the English language was discussed extensively with Ali John Comegys. I am grateful to both of them. Finally, I wish to thank KAZI Publications, Inc. for believing in this work and encouraging me to complete it.

Morality, the Law and the Way

Morality in Islamic culture has its origin in religion. It has developed exclusively within that framework. Based on the beliefs of the traditional Islamic society as revealed in the Quran, God is of an ethical nature and acts upon the human being in an ethical way. This creates a responsibility on the part of the human being who has been given the trust of nature to respond in an ethical way, as well. The human response in the monotheistic tradition is through religion in its universal sense as containing both a Law and a Way. In such a traditional society, the Law contains the principles and practices which regulate human behavior whether it be as an individual or as a member of a society while the Way concentrates on the inner meaning within things.

The basic principle through which the Way becomes operative is that there is a hidden meaning in all things. Everything created has an outer and inner meaning; every external form has a complementary, inner reality which is its hidden, eternal essence. While the external form emphasizes the quantitative aspect, the most apparent and obvious form of a thing, the internal essence reflects the qualitative aspect. In order to know a thing in its completeness, one must seek both the outward form and the inner reality. It is in its inner essence that the eternal beauty of every object resides.[1]

The relationship is perhaps best expressed through the metaphor of a circle. The Law is as the circumference, the Way as radii leading to the center, Reality. Without the circumference, there would be no Way; without the Way there would be no need for the radii; without the center there would be no understanding of Reality.

Both the ethics of the Law and the ethics of the Way respond to the innate function of counseling to the positive and preventing the development of the negative in both this life and the next. The difference is that one is the

3

container and the other the contained. It is the qualitative, inward "all that is contained," quality to which the Way relates. Without it, the human being is only the physical form yet without the physical form there would be nothing to "contain."

A line from Rūmī expresses this when he says, "We are the flute, our music is Thine's." Our outer form, regulated by the Law, is as a reed flute through which passes the breath. The quality of the construction of the inside of the flute is as relevant to the music produced as the outside form. Both are essential if there is to be music. What the inside or qualitative aspect of the flute wants to be in order to produce harmonic sounds dictates the outside shape of the flute. The same is true of the human form. While the Law concentrates on the ethics of the container, the Way concentrates on those of the contained. The ethics of the Way, then, are in addition to those of the Law and not that one can be substituted for the other.

The ethics of the Law and the Way, on the other hand, are interconnected through what is known as spiritual hermeneutics (ta'wil). Spiritual hermeneutics has two basic requirements: a Divine Law revealed to a divinely chosen Messenger and a Way or gnosis (ma'rifah). While the Law deals with the horizontal axis, the material plane, the quantitative aspects of self, the sensible, the Way is concerned with the Vertical Axis, the spiritual, the qualitative, the intelligible realm of self. Spiritual hermeneutics is the bridge over which one intellectually passes between the quantitative and the qualitative. While the quantitative appears in the sensible world and is capable of direct and objective experience, the qualitative can only be known indirectly by the effects that it produces. While the quantitative speaks through the Signs of outer forms *"upon the horizons,"* (41:53), the qualitative speaks through Signs of meaning *"within themselves"* (41:53).

Spiritual hermeneutics interprets the Signs through a

language of symbolism. Inner meaning can only be understood in a time that transcends history because Essence,
the Divinity in the Absolute sense, is neither time nor
space bound. It is to this timeless, spaceless world that
Signs of inner meaning relate, Signs which are vital to the
spiritual warrior who recognizes the importance of both
outer form and inner meaning.

Clearly there are Signs (āyah, verses) of the Quran
which need a formal, moral interpretation as conditions
for the trustee of nature to have such as the fact that eating
pork is forbidden along with the taking of intoxicants or
any kind or gambling. In the same way, things that are
obligatory like the daily ritual prayers, fasting during the
month of Ramadan, the giving of alms to charity and the
once in a lifetime pilgrimage to Makkah, if one has the
economic means to do so, all fall within that which is
morally obligatory upon the monotheist (ḥanīf).

When the spiritual warrior looks to the stories in the
Quran, some of them can be clearly explained by the Law
while others fall outside a formal interpretation. The Law
deals with the outer form and not the meaning held within
the form. In not attending to the meaning, it also leaves
out the eternal beauty which resides in each form. As the
Quran says about the Messenger, *"He has a beautiful character so follow him"* (33:21). As the Messenger says, "God is
beautiful," and "God loves beauty."

For instance, the Quran says that Asiyah, the foster-
mother of Moses, rebelled against her husband, the
Pharaoh, because of his tyranny and injustice. The
Pharaoh calling for the death of all new born male children is clearly a forbidden (ḥarām) act according to the
Law. Following the command to counsel to the good or
positive and prevent the development of the negative,
Asiyah was acting within the Law to rebel against him and
to seek refuge in God from the Pharaoh. Instead of remaining an idolater as the Pharaoh was, she chose the way of

nature originated by God (*fiṭrat Allāh*) and became a follower of Moses, a monotheist (*ḥanīf*), realizing as she did that in the monotheistic system each person is accountable for their own deeds. A wife cannot say that she could not obey the Commands because her husband would not allow it nor vice versa.

Ethical responses at the level of the Law are dealt with in Islamic jurisprudence in determining what is right from what is wrong according to the Commands of the Commander-in-Chief, Almighty God, whose orders are followed by the moral-seeker. Jurisprudence (*fiqh*) divides all actions into five categories of moral response:

1. *Wājib*: Obligatory duties which are absolutely necessary, the neglect of which is punishable by the Law.

2. *Mustahab*: Recommended duties which are not obligatory. The performing of them is rewarded while the neglect of performance of them is not punishable.

3. *Ja'iz*: Acts that are allowed that may or may not be done. Neither rewards nor punishments are incurred.

4. *Makrūh*: Acts that are disapproved, the non-performance of which results in rewards while the doing of them is not punishable.

5. *Ḥarām*: Forbidden acts are forbidden by God and therefore punishable by the Law.

Examples of past peoples that cannot be explained by the ethics of the Law alone can be seen in some of the stories of Abraham and the story of Moses and Khidr. Abraham, founder of spiritual chivalry, asks the Lord to let him see how the Lord brings back to life something that is dead.

> *And when Abraham asked God, 'My Lord! Show me how You give life to the dead!'*
> *God said, 'What! Do you not believe?'*
> *Abraham said, 'Yes, but so my heart may be at ease.'*
> *Then God said, 'Take four birds...Train them to follow you. Then place a part of them on every mountain. Then call*

them. They will come flying to you...' (2:260)

How does the ethics of the Law explain Abraham's answer to *"What! Do you not believe?"* by his saying, *"Yes, but so my heart may be at ease?"* The ethics of the Law, the formal aspect of things, does not regulate the heart.

The story of Moses and Khidr related in the Quran is another example and perhaps one of the most direct indications of the presence of the Way as the inner dimension of the Islamic Tradition. Moses is promised a meeting with someone who is more knowledgeable than he. Traditional commentators say that the person he meets is Khidr, the inner guide. The story of their meeting and the unfolding of events are described further on. Here it should be noted that there are Signs as that of Khidr which speak to another kind of ethics—the ethics of the Way.

The ethical response at the level of the Way is to learn to read the Signs according to the Quran, *"We shall show them Our Signs upon the horizons and within themselves until it is clear to them that it is the Real (the Truth),"* (41:53) for it is through Signs that the Presence of God is made known. Learning to read the Signs is part of the duties and obligations of being His trustee of nature and of the self. This is what the moral healers struggle to become as they transform into spiritual warriors moving towards the model of spiritual chivalry.

PART II
SPIRITUAL CHIVALRY

CHAPTER 1: THE GOAL

Spiritual chivalry (*futuwwah*) is best known in the West in an historic context. What is least understood is its inner connection to traditional Islam. It is part of the fabric of the traditional Muslim whose life did not make the pages of history but whose belief in the One God (*fiṭrat Allāh*) was woven into the very fabric of his or her existence manifested as service to others before any consideration was given to self. This model is alive and well in a traditional society—one that follows both a Law and a Way—of which Islam, in particular, in its inner dimension or Sufism, is the present example.

Sufism can be approached from various perspectives while the sources for any or all perspectives are the same. These two sources include first, the revelation of the Quran. The Quran had been recorded by scribes at the moment of revelation and collected in the form of the present chapters (*surahs*) two years after the death of the Messenger and compiled in its present form by the major scribe twelve years after the Messenger's death. The second source is the sayings and customs of the Messenger Muhammad known as the *sunnah*. The *sunnah* had been recorded by those who directly bore witness to the Messenger, his words and actions and are recorded in books on the Traditions (*aḥadilh*, sing. *ḥadith*).

A traditional Sufi defines spiritual chivalry in the following way:

> Spiritual chivalry (*futuwwah*) consists in the manifestation of the Light of the original nature (*fiṭrat Allāh*) and its gaining mastery over the negative effects within the physical form. All positive traits become manifest within the self and all negative qualities disappear... The human being perseveres in these affairs until the force of the animal self (passions) is broken, its

strength and negative traits are overcome and firmness becomes the person's second nature...Then all kinds of **temperance** and **courage** become firmly rooted in him. All the varieties of **wisdom** and **justice** become manifest in him in actuality.[1]

Another Sufi points out, "The follower of spiritual chivalry is called a spiritual warrior *(fatā)*. It is a person who resists self-will (the passions) by engaging in the greater struggle *(jihād al-akbar)*."[2]

Moral healing is the first stage to attain according to the Way. It is said that the Prophet Seth was the first to describe the inner Way for the human being. His followers wore a cloak. As the weight of this cloak became difficult to bear, Prophet Abraham initiated the way of spiritual chivalry. That is, the complete stages of the Way are difficult to bear and few manage to complete the stages in their lifetime, but if they at least complete the stage of spiritual chivalry, they will have prepared themselves for the position of trustee for which they were created.[3]

To have morally healed through the self-help method of self-examination as delineated in the Sign of "the Presence of God" is to have centered the self in wisdom (faith in the One God), courage (trust in the One God), temperance (charity towards God's creatures) and justice (putting Reality in Its proper perspective). This is considered to be moral goodness *(murūwwah)*. Proof of the latter positive trait, that is, succeeding in putting Reality in Its proper place, is only attained if one benefits another person and that person confirms the presence of fairness and justice. This is to attain the stage of spiritual chivalry *(futuwwah)*.

NATURE ORIGINATED BY GOD

The goal of spiritual chivalry is to transfer the Light of

nature originated by God (*fiṭrat Allāh*) from potentiality to actuality. This nature originated by God is referred to in the Quran in the following verse,

> *Then set your face towards the religion of monotheism (al-dīn ḥanīfan) in natural devotion to the Truth of nature originated by God (fiṭrat Allāh) in which He originated the people; no change can there be (by anyone else) in this creation of God* (30:30).

In the view of spiritual chivalry, the human being is not born in a state of original sin but in a state originated by God, the state of worshipping the One God. This natural disposition to the worship of the One God is a nature which has the potential to sense the order, balance, harmony and equilibrium in the universe. The human acceptance of this nature originated by God comes from the covenant which the human being accepted when God formed it.

> *And when your Lord took the seed of the children of Adam from their loins and [asked], 'Am I not your Lord?' and they bore witness, 'Yea, we do bear witness...'* so that they not respond on the Day of Judgment by saying, *'We were unaware of this'* (7:172).

This covenant and the following trust are aspects of the Divine Spirit within which God blew only into the human form. It is what gives meaning to the human being.

Having accepted the covenant at formation, as part of one's *fiṭrat Allāh*, the human being was then given the trust of nature.

> *We offered the trust to the heavens and the earth and the mountains, but they refused to carry it and were afraid of it, and the human being carried it* (33:72).

have been sent in the form of Prophets. The Prophets remind the human being of their duties and obligations and the rewards or punishments for performing or not. The Reminderers remind through revelation. Revelation is of two kinds: First, the created order is itself a universal revelation of the Presence of God. Second, because the human being was created with consciousness of self, this aspect of consciousness needs a different kind of reminder, a different kind of revelation, an additional kind of guidance and that is the revelation that the Prophets as Reminderers bring.

A Tradition which follows from the Sign of the human being being born from a nature originated by God (*fiṭrat Allāh*), which is the religion of monotheism (*al-dīn ḥanīfan*), is: "Every creature that is born has an original nature (*fiṭrat*) of submission (*islām*) but their fathers and mothers cause them to deviate."

The spiritual warrior recognizes from this that the human being, as a species, has been created with the preparedness to accept religion as submission to God's Will (*islām*) and if left alone and to itself in its natural state, it will choose that very way unless external factors cause it to deviate from its natural way.

Religion, then, is innate. It is a Way of life, a truth within human nature. Thus the Quran says that that which Noah had is called religion and its name is submission (*islām*); that which Abraham had is called religion and its name is submission (*islām*); and that which Moses and Jesus and all the other rightful Prophets had is called religion and its name is submission (*islām*) (42:13) because there is no distinction among the Prophets as the Sign says,

We believe in God and that which has been sent down on us and sent down on Abraham and Ishmael, Isaac and Jacob, and the Tribes, and in that which was given to Moses and Jesus, and the Prophets

We believe in God and that which has been sent down on us and sent down on Abraham and Ishmael, Isaac and Jacob, and the Tribes, and in that which was given to Moses and Jesus, and the Prophets from their Lord; we make no division between any of them, and to Him we surrender (muslim). If any one desires a religion other than submission (to God's Will, islām) never will it be accepted of him... (3:84-85).

The words *fiṭrat Allāh* are similar in meaning in the Quran to *sibghāh* and *ḥanīf*. *Sibghāh* is referred to where it says, *"God's coloring (sibghāh Allāh) and Who is better than God's coloring; while Him (alone) do we worship"* (2:138). It refers to a kind of color which God uses, a color which God has painted into the fabric of creation, referring to religion. This is the Divine Coloring through which the Hand of Truth colored the very fabric of the creation of the human being.

In regard to the word *ḥanīf*, a Sign says, *"Abraham was neither a Jew nor a Christian, but a monotheist (ḥanīf,), a submitter to God's Will (muslim)..."* (3:67). He followed the religion of monotheism, following the natural predisposition to which God predisposed humanity. The Quran says a person has only one *fiṭrat* and that *fiṭrat* is the person's religion and that natural religion is submission to the Will of God (*islām*).

The word monotheist (*ḥanīf*) describes a person who follows the "true religion." This is deep-rooted within the self in the nature originated by God— submission to God's Will. This submission in the monotheist is absolute and the antithesis of worshipping more than One God. Abraham reconfirmed this message in his words and actions as one who submits to God's Will (*muslim*), a monotheist (*ḥanīf*).

To be a monotheist is to have the desire and inclination towards the Truth, the Real. A monotheist, then, is a truth-seeker, reality-seeker, seeker of God, seeker of unity. This is the basis for the spiritual warrior actualizing the moral reasonableness of a religiously cultured monotheist (*hilm*). It is the nurturing process which changes this natural state by covering over the inner Light of the nature originated by God with ignorance of Reality. The ignorance (*jahl*) is manifested in many ways as we will see among which are ungratefulness for life and its blessings (*kufr*), disbelief in the One Reality (*kufr*), belief in a multiple of realities instead of the One (*shirk*), or pretending to believe in the One Reality with one's tongue but denying It with one's deeds (*nifāq*).

THE LIGHT

Spiritual chivalry as initiated by Prophet Abraham has as its goal the actualization of the nature by which God originated the human being (*fitrat Allāh*) and this nature is seen as an inner Light located at the center of self. When this Light illuminates the heart, the heart turns towards the spiritual. Without the inner Light of this nature originated by God, the heart is in a state of ignorance of Reality. Through the nurturing process, this inner Light becomes veiled. The veiling of the Light of the nature originated by God, in turn, veils the spiritual potential of the heart. Two major factors which cause the inner Light to dim are the domination of the self by the idol/ego within and the tendency of the self to forget Reality. The idol/ego is the animal self attached to the material world, making the same demands on self that God does. Attachment to one's ego—desires for the material world as opposed to the Light which opens onto the spiritual world—little by little, bit by bit, veils the possibility of the heart turning towards the spiritual world. This veiling of the spiritual heart increases through forgetfulness of Reality showing the need for Reminders and Reminderers.

This nature originated by Allah is veiled by anything that takes the spiritual warrior away from the remembrance of God. The biological state in which the individual finds self may be the veil where the natural elements combine in an imbalanced way, or it may be the society or culture in which one grows up which veils one from this inner Light. The spiritual warrior spends no time looking for the reason for the veiling concentrating rather on the fact that it has become veiled and that the only way out is to engage in struggle with the idol within.

GRACE

This Light can also be seen as Divine Grace. For the spiritual warrior, there is Grace wherever God is Present. Grace results from the contact of the human spirit with the Divine Spirit. The human spirit is an aspect of the Divine Spirit working within and influencing the self. Grace is always there but not always operative in full measure unless the self is "prepared" to receive it. "Preparedness" is attained through moral healing of the self. Once the self has morally healed, Divine Grace may be "revealed" to the self.

A spiritual warrior describes Grace in the following way:

Grace is God's loving kindness and mercy and turning towards Him. The beginning of the greater struggle, the spiritual struggle, is itself the Call of God. The help given to enable the spiritual warrior to return to Him is one of the greatest Gifts of God.[4]

To an early Sufi the Grace of God is a Light supernatural (*nūr al-qulūb*) whereby the hearts of people are illuminated.

Nothing is more hard upon moral imbalance than Light but the Light is only an illumination of the spiritual aspect of the heart if the servant is awake and alive to it. When he is neglectful, his heart lies dormant, in potential, in darkness. The Light within is extinguished and nothing is more pleasing to Iblis than to have darkness surround the spiritual because of the dimming to extinction of the Light.[5]

Wrongdoing, self-centeredness, egotism and/or self-worship, pride, arrogance, haughtiness, attachment to worldly things, extravagance, miserliness, envy, greed and so forth restrain the self from moral healing. Only when these negative traits have been overcome and the will has surrendered or submitted to a higher Will can Grace have free course. Those who hear the Call and respond attempting to morally heal through constant self-examination have "opened their hearts" to His Grace. God then freely gives that which He is always ready to give. A Divine Tradition[6] confirms this view:

> Oh son of Adam, if you draw near to Me by half a span, I will approach you by a span and if you approach Me by a span, I will approach you by a cubit, and if you approach Me by a cubit, I will approach you by a fathom, and if you do come to Me walking, I will come to you in haste.[7]

KNOWLEDGE

Every Way emphasizes an aspect of the Truth and for Islam the emphasis is upon this inner Light in its aspect of knowledge. With the Light of Grace as its Source, knowledge is integrated into the principle of Unity or the Oneness of God which runs as the Vertical Axis through every mode of knowledge and being. The source for knowledge and its development in traditional Islamic sciences is the Quran and the customs and sayings of God's Messenger Muhammad. The Quran is Itself the Logos or Word of God revealed to the Messenger Muhammad over a period of twenty-three years. It is the natural unfolding of creation containing the archetypes of all things within it. Each of the 6600 and some verses are called "Signs" as is everything in the universe including the human self within according to the "Sign," "*We shall show them Our Signs upon the horizons and within themselves until it is clear to them that it is the Real (the Truth)*" (41:53).

With these concepts of the Quran and the *sunnah* as extensions of nature where the cosmic and natural order overflow with Divine Grace or *barakah*, one as the Word of God and the other as the most perfect model in following the Word of God, the human being's relation with nature is one of a sense of unity and oneness. Through knowledge gained in contemplating nature in all its facets, the human being learns to read the Signs and act upon them thus becoming the channel of Divine Grace.

> The human being sees in nature what he is himself and penetrates into the inner meaning of nature only on the condition of being able to delve into the inner depths of his own being and to cease to lie merely on the periphery of his being.[8]

The Light of nature originated by God is also seen as knowledge of Reality. The spiritual warrior, seeing the real self by the Light originated by God within, perceives that all human individuality is nothing but appearance, illusion. This knowledge, unlike knowledge gained through sense perception, remains as an everlasting gift with the spiritual warrior.

CHAPTER 2: THE HEART

The word for heart in Arabic is *qalb*. It is defined as "reversal, overturn, transformation, change" and "alteration, fluctuation, variableness, inconstancy."[1] As its nature is to fluctuate, it is referred to by different names depending upon which direction it is facing. It may be called the soul (animal self, the passions), spirit and/or reason. Ibn al-'Arabī, however, makes it clear that it can only refer to reason if reason is defined as "that which is delimited by fluctuation so that it never ceases undergoing transformation..."[2] This will be important for us to note later.

Sufis regard the heart as the essence of the self, an immaterial principle which controls the conscious life of the human being by which Reality is perceived and interpreted. When seen as self, it symbolizes the whole human personality or personality in its wholeness. It is the heart which makes the human being human. It is that which separates the human being from all other creatures. It is that which enables the human being to have knowledge of God, to accept or reject His counseling to the positive and prevention of the negative. It is the point of union where the body and self unite, where the physical meets the spiritual, the place of the meeting of the two seas. It is the only thing that God wants from His servants as an early Sufi writes, "God only desires their hearts from His servants and their physical members will follow their hearts."[3]

While the actions of a human being's physical members are under control of the heart in terms of directing them to the positive or the negative, the actions of the heart include the human being's motivation for outward conduct. Motivation includes the processes of thinking, feeling and actions. These include the use of positive or negative traits, the positive traits falling within the cate-

gories of wisdom, courage, temperance and justice, receptivity to positive psychological states and the attainment
of spiritual states.

The heart is compared to the Kabah, the earthly temple, making it "the noblest house in the believer."[4] It is
also said to be the Throne of God in the microcosm. This
refers to a sacred Tradition, "My earth and My heaven
embrace Me not, but the heart of My believing servant
does embrace Me."[5] The heart "embraces God" through
knowledge of God, knowledge that comes from the inner
Light of the nature originated by God.

The heart is said in a Tradition to dwell between the
two fingers of the All-Merciful. "The hearts of all the children of Adam are like a single heart between two of the
fingers of the All-Merciful. He turns it wherever He
desires.[6] The All-Merciful according to the Quran "*sat
upon the Throne*" (20:5) and God's mercy "*embraces all
things*" (7:156). The only other quality which embraces all
things is knowledge, "*Our Lord, You embrace all things in
Mercy and in Knowledge*" (40:7).[7]

The heart, then, as the Throne of God, is the place for
knowledge of the Reality. This is the spiritual and not the
physical heart yet there are similarities. In a Tradition, the
Messenger asks: "Within the human being there is a fleshy
fragment and when it is corrupt, the body is corrupt and
when it is sound, the body is sound. Is it not the heart?"[8]
In regard to the spiritual aspect of the heart, he said,
"When a person makes his inward self sound, God will
make his outward conduct sound; when the secret life has
been purified, God will purify the outward manifestation
thereof."[9]

The heart is like a mirror which functions as such
when it is brightly polished and has been freed of all rust
of wrongdoing or negative traits. The Quran says, "*...But
on their hearts is the stain of the (ill) which they do!*" (83:14)"

It is through the heart that one gains access to knowledge of this world and the next. As Hujwīrī says,

> When a person feels desire and passion, he turns to
> the heart in order that it may guide him to the lower
> soul which is the seat of falsehood and when he finds
> the evidence of gnosis, he also turns to the heart in
> order that it may guide him to the spirit which is the
> source of Truth and Reality.[10]

THE GREATER STRUGGLE

Whereas the mystical dimension is most often described as a journey from God to God, spiritual chivalry, the moral dimension, is described as a struggle, the greater struggle (*jihād al-akbar*), the struggle within. This struggle takes place between two basic aspects of our nature: our animal self known as "the passions," (*nafs ammārah*) which through nurture develops into the idol/ego within, and our ability to reason. The winner in the struggle controls the heart. If reason wins the struggle, the self becomes morally healed by gaining the ability to direct the heart towards the Lord because of the presence of the Light that is now illuminated. If the passions win, the aspiring spiritual warrior has lost both this world and the next.

Reason, as an aspect of spirit within, needs to be developed at three levels: between the animal and spiritual self within (psychoethics), between the self and others (socioethics) and between the self and God (theoethics). At the level of psychoethics, it means to be centered, balanced in reason, reason ruling over the passions. At the level of socioethics it means to deal with others in a fair and just manner, putting others and their needs before self. In regard to the spiritual warrior's relationship with God, it means "to put things in their proper place," "to accept Reality as Trust-Giver and self as trustee." When the spiritual warrior operates on these three levels in the manner described, the person is morally healed.

The greater struggle takes place for the heart as it fluctuates this way and that. It is the spirit or reason understood as Ibn al-'Arabī defines it that turns the heart towards the spiritual. The idol within follows the "passions," the animal aspect consisting of an over use or misuse of feelings (to preserve the species) and actions (to preserve the individual). While these two functions are a necessary part of the life of the human species, their overuse or misuse result in the animal aspect ruling the self. It is then that they are referred to as the passions. The domination of the self by the passions results in the desires of the passions becoming an idol within. It makes endless demands upon the self including the demand to obedience and constant admiration. As Suhrāwārdī explains it:

> The animal self makes the same demands of obedience and admiration on the human being as does God. It is a delicate matter lodged within this mold of the body. The animal self is the substratum of negative qualities. The spirit is the mine of positive and the animal self is the mine of the negative. The intellect is the army of the spirit and success which is granted by Allah is its reinforcement. Capricious desire is the army of the animal self and failure is its reinforcement.[11]

The struggle is to "destroy the idol" within. This process begins with the realization that the idol within is a false idol. The inappropriate desires of the passions have to be controlled by reason. It is a painful struggle within the self to strengthen one's sense of humility before God and His creatures, to subdue the passions to serve God's purposes and not the desires of the self. It is to lose the false aspect of self in order to find the true self as it was created to be. It is dying before you die, dying in order to live. As Rūmī asks, "Can bread give strength unless it be broken?"

The heart symbolizes the human reality. When it turns towards and fluctuates towards desires of the idol/ego, it is called the passions or *nafs ammārah*. When it turns towards moral healing, it is called the spirit or reason (*nafs lawwāmah*). It is in this capacity that it is then the place for the knowledge of Reality. It is then the quality "of knowing God and witnessing the beauty of His Presence."

The struggle within, the greater struggle (*jihād al-akbar*), between the idol/ego and the spirit, both aspects of human nature, is more easily won if the nurturing process is a positive one. A positive nurturing process is one that reinforces reason as opposed to one that over or under or even totally undevelops one's natural ability to reason. According to traditional psychoethics, no matter what the nurturing process has been, the awareness of the need to morally heal is itself God's Calling of the person and the time to begin.

Through moral healing, the spiritual warrior learns to assume the Names of Beauty, qualities through which the One God manifests Self. Learning that the One God is the Merciful, the Compassionate, the Forgiving, the Acceptor of Repentance and so forth, causes the spiritual warrior to rise above nature and nurture—whatever the obstacle be—in the greater struggle to morally heal the self. In other words, nothing precludes victory in this greater struggle except God's Will. If the spiritual warrior were to say to self, "God is Just. I am among His people. He has given me the possibility of becoming His trustee of nature. He wants me to earn that trusteeship. To earn it, I have to morally heal so that my society can morally heal," that person has heard the Call.

God's Will is seen as operative within the processes of nature. The spiritual warrior consciously engages in a battle between nature as the animal self and nature as reason, an aspect of the spirit within. Both of these are conceived as aspects of God's Will. That is why guidance through revelation is essential so that the human being is guided in the right direction, oriented towards the spirit within rather than the animal or passions within. As the spiritual warrior goes through the struggle, he or she may conclude that the animal self is also an aspect of God's Will operating within and therefore rationalize that it is to be played out forgetting that there is a spiritual side to self that is also an aspect of God's Will operating within which is as an inner Light. That Light, as guidance through revelation describes, becomes veiled by the animal self and can only be unveiled if the spirit within is victorious in the greater struggle. The heart of those who repeatedly choose to remain in ignorance (*jahl*) of Reality may be further veiled by God or even further He may cause disease to appear in their heart.

Spiritual warriors, learning to read God's Signs, undertakes the battle, accepts the challenge with the knowledge that there is no guarantee of success, learns to read the Signs, with the knowledge that any success belongs to God. Motivated by a deep love for God, the potential hero (*fatā javānmard*) or heroine (*fatāt, javānmard*), spiritual warrior, moves through the traditional stages on the return to their divinely originated nature to unveil the spiritual aspect of their heart.

The return for the spiritual warrior, these retracing of one's steps back to one's original nature which is none other than the "true religion," the worship of the One God, follows a well-trodden process. It is a process which all of nature follows but which the human being must choose and that is moral reasonableness. Nature is based in moral reasonableness through a mystical participation with the divinity, the Creator. The human being, on the other hand, has to make the choice, has to commit self and accept the responsibility of this choice to attain the moral reasonableness of religiously cultured monotheist (*ḥilm*).

MORAL REASONABLENESS OF A RELIGIOUSLY CULTURED MONOTHEIST

While each level of spiritual chivalry has its own particular manifestations, there is also a universal characteristic or quality which is made manifest in the spiritual warrior. The spiritual warrior is then described as having the moral reasonableness of a religiously cultured monotheist. A person who is called ḥalīm, the noun form of hilm, is the description of someone who has attained the stage of murūwwah or moral goodness.

The entire Quran is described as having this ethic.

There is constant counsel to kindness towards others (iḥsān) with emphasis on being just. Oppression and wrongful violence (ẓulm) are forbidden and one is repeatedly exhorted to command to good and prevent evil. Pride and arrogance are condemned while patience and forbearance are encouraged. Moral reasonableness is a positive and active quality which the spiritual warrior uses as a powerful weapon to prevent the self from being impulsive and hasty. It allows the spiritual warrior to develop patience and forbearance. He (or she) is able to restrain the self from striking back when provoked even though one clearly has the physical ability to do so. It requires constant consciousness and self-examination to remain calm in adverse situations, to forgive one's enemies and show gentleness towards them. It is the spiritual warrior—calm with a balanced mind, self-controlled who exhibits steadiness of judgment. The state is expressed through what is called dignity of manner and behavior (waqār).[12]

This quality of moral reasonableness brings balance and a sense of centeredness to the spiritual warrior which is manifested in three relationships: that of the spiritual warrior towards his or her Lord (theoethics); that of the spiritual warrior towards creation (socioethics); and that of the spiritual warrior towards self (psychoethics). In the first type of relationship, the spiritual warrior has attained certain knowledge of Reality; in the second type of relationship, the spiritual warrior puts others above self; and in the third type of relationship, the spiritual warrior has actualized his or her nature originated by God, which, in turn, has allowed the inner Light to illuminate the spiritual aspect of the heart. Proof of this process, which is to have been victorious in the greater struggle, is manifested in four positive traits: wisdom (belief in the One God), courage (trust in the One God), temperance (charity towards others) and justice (having the ability to put Reality in Its proper place).

THEOETHICS

At the level of theoethics, the appearance of the moral reasonableness of a religiously cultured monotheist allows the spiritual warrior to experience the ethical nature of God as Trust-Giver to his or her trusteeship. God describes Himself in the Quran through His Most Beautiful Names which are essential to Divine Ethics. One of these Names mentioned in the Quran is Ḥalīm. The entire revelation speaks to the spiritual warrior's in terms of moral reasonableness. Spiritual warriors see that God forgives wrongdoings and is gentle towards them while having the power to do otherwise. Spiritual warriors know they have been forgiven when they no longer repeat wrongdoing from which they have repented and asked for forgiveness. Spiritual warriors see that God is the Forbearing and the Patient, the Merciful and the Compassionate while clearly having the power to punish and retaliate. Spiritual warriors then learn the same ethical response in dealing with self and others. They learn to give to others what they themselves need (ithār). This is to model their behavior on the process of creation itself.

With the world view of the spiritual warrior of religion in its most universal sense, the response is an ethical-religious response. The clearest example of spiritual chivalry at the level of the Divinity is creation itself. It is considered to be the greatest act of charity for there was no need to do it.

He only brings the cosmos into existence for the sake of the cosmos, as an act of charity (ithār) toward it in spite of the fact that He alone possesses Being. This is spiritual chivalry itself.[13]

To follow the model of spiritual chivalry is to manifest a portion of the Divine Name, the Creator. Creation, in the Islamic perspective, however, is not considered to be a one time event whereafter the Creator removed Self from the world but an ongoing process whereby at every moment, with every breath, we die and are born again.

In describing theoethics, Anṣārī says,

Spiritual chivalry towards God is to strive in servanthood with all one's strength. There are three Signs for the spiritual warrior: never tire of seeking knowledge, never cease remembering God and finding companions among good people.[14]

For the spiritual warrior the response is to see self as the servant ('abd) of the Lord (rabb). As God is the Absolute, the only human response is that of complete submission (islām), humbleness and humility (islam). Through worship ('ibādah), the servant serves God as a servant As the Quran commands,

*Lord of the heavens and the earth and of all that is
between them. So worship Him and be constant and patient
in His worship. Do you know of any who is worthy of the
same Name as He?* (19:65).

SOCIOETHICS

Social life falls under the rules and regulations of a certain set of moral principles which form the brotherhoods and sisterhoods of spiritual chivalry. Spiritual warriors act with justice towards the members of their community because God's actions are just. A Sign says, *"The Word changes not before Me and I do not the least injustice to My servants"* (50:29). Spiritual warriors should not wrong members of their community because God does not wrong anybody even by *'the weight of an ant'* (4:49) or *'by a single date-thread'* (4:40).

Spiritual warriors are told,

> You ask for nothing extra for yourself and you see yourself as not having any rights. You do this in three stages: first, leave aside quarreling, overlook the slips that others make and forget their wrongs. The next step is to draw close to those who distance themselves from you, honor those who wrong you and make excuses for those who offend you. You do this by being generous not by holding yourself back. It comes from letting go not by bearing it with patience.[15]

Spiritual warriors learn three sayings of the Messenger on friendship. "The human being is in the religion of his friend, therefore you should consider carefully whom you befriend." "A person who mixes with people and endures their evil is superior to one who does not mix with people." "There is no benefit in him who does not befriend others and is not befriended."[16]

PSYCHOETHICS

The third relationship develops psychoethics. The spiritual warrior then engages in a spiritual struggle with the self to overcome the false ego and to develop the moral reasonableness of a religiously cultured monotheist by manifesting the first stage of spiritual chivalry, that of moral goodness (*murūwwah*).

Through the development of this level of ethics, spiritual warriors are described as having attained the moral reasonableness of a religiously cultured monotheist. They forsake their own will in all things and disregard their own private self-love; they refuse to gratify natural desires before consulting with reason; they acknowledge that they are nothing and worse than animals; they promptly obey God in their own heart and other human beings in outward affairs; they cease to become entangled in unnecessary things and superfluous cares; they allow the deeds and words of others to pass by unheard and yield to no rash judgment; they are unduly moved neither by the praise nor the blame of other human beings; they bear any injury, adversity or misery they may encounter within or without with forbearance; they indulge in not even a slight and passing complaint; and they entertain a sense of charity for all human beings.

CHAPTER 3: SPIRITUAL MODELS

In keeping with the spiritual hermeneutics of the Way, the spiritual warrior uses models in a different way than normally represented. A model for the spiritual warrior is anyone who manifests the moral reasonableness of a religiously cultured monotheist (*ḥilm*). Essentially it refers to anyone who has morally healed. While the outer accomplishments of the person are important whether or not the person strived in God's Cause, it is the inner dimension which is emphasized in spiritual chivalry, the outer expressions of inner meaning.

The main source for the models is the Quran. The Chapter of the Cave (*Surah Kahf*), for instance, contains the story of the Companions of the Cave as well as stories related to the Messenger Muhammad, Prophet Abraham, Moses and Dhul Qarnayn, the 'man with two horns'. The stories are interpreted through spiritual hermeneutics, each one of these models symbolizing the struggle within. The stories are understood at two levels by the spiritual warrior. First, as outward models and second as Divine guidance for the inward struggle, the greater struggle with the idol within.

As an example, we will take the story of Moses and Khidr and that of Dhul Qarnayn. The outward story of Moses and Khidr is presented first and then we will embark upon its inward meaning for the spiritual warrior described by Ibn al-'Arabī.

MOSES AND KHIDR

And when Moses said to his attendant (fatā, Joshua), 'I will not give up until I reach the meeting of the two seas even though it may take me many years.' Then, when they reached the junction (where the two seas meet), they forgot their fish and it took its way into the sea. When they had passed over, (Moses) said to his attendant (Joshua), 'Bring us our food. Indeed, we are exhausted by our journey.' (Joshua) said, 'You see! When we rested near the bedrock, I forgot the fish—and

it was Satan that made me forget so that I should not remem-
ber it—and so it took its way into the sea in a marvelous man-
ner.' (Moses) said, 'This is what we were seeking!' and so
they returned upon their tracks, retracing them.

Then they found one of Our servants unto whom We had
given mercy from Us (Khidr) and We had taught him knowl-
edge proceeding from Us. Moses said to (Khidr), 'May I fol-
low you so that you teach me of what you have been taught,
right judgment?' (Khidr) said, 'Assuredly you will not be able
to bear with me patiently. How could you bear patiently that
which you have never encompassed in your knowledge?'
(Moses) said, 'Yet you shall find me, if God will, patient and I
shall not rebel against you in anything.' (Khidr) said, 'Then if
you follow me, do not question me on anything until I myself
introduce the mention of it to you.'

So they departed until when they embarked upon a ship.
(Khidr) made a hole in (the bottom of the ship). (Moses) said,
'What, have you made a hole in it so as to drown its passen-
gers? You have indeed done a grievous thing.' (Khidr) said,
'Did I not say that you could never bear with me patiently?'
(Moses) said, 'Do not take me to task that I forgot, neither ask
me to do a thing too difficult.'

So they departed until when they met a lad. (Khidr) slew
him. (Moses) said, 'What, have you slain an innocent soul
and that not to retaliate for a soul slain? You have indeed
done a horrible thing.' (Khidr) said, 'Did I not say that you
could never bear with me patiently?' (Moses) said, 'If I ques-
tion you on anything after this, then do not keep company
with me. You have already experienced excuse sufficient on
my part.'

So they departed until when they reached the people of a
city and they asked the people for food but they refused to
receive them hospitably. There they found a wall about to
tumble down and so (Khidr) set it up. (Moses) said, 'If you
had wished, you could have taken a wage for that.' (Khidr)
said, 'This is the parting between me and you. Now I will tell
you the interpretation of that which you could not bear
patiently. As for the ship, it belonged to certain poor men who

toiled upon the sea. I desired to damage it for behind them there was a king who was seizing every ship with brutal force. As for the lad, his parents were believers and we were afraid he would impose on them insolence and unbelief so we desired that their Lord should give to them in exchange one better than he in purity and nearer in tenderness. As for the wall, it belonged to two orphan lads in the city and under it was a treasure belonging to them. Their father was a righteous man and your Lord desired that they should come of age and then bring forth their treasure as a mercy from your Lord. I did it not of my own bidding. This is the interpretation of that which you could not bear patiently' (18:57-83).

The spiritual hermeneutics of the story follows:

<u>And when Moses said</u>, this is the outer explanation of what was told (in the Quran and earlier scriptures) and there is no denying miracles herein. As for the inward meaning, "And <u>when</u> the heart," said to the self at the time when the heart and the self clung to the body because of physical desires and demands, "<u>I will not give up,</u>" the spiritual quest, I will not stop walking or traveling towards my spiritual goal, "<u>until I reach the junction of the two seas,</u>" the two worlds, the world of the self and the world of the body, that is, the two waters of the sweet and the salty in the human being in the station in the heart "<u>even though it may take me many years.</u>"

Then, <u>when they reached the junction (where the two seas meet)</u>, the place where physical and psychic forces meet in a combined form, <u>they forgot their fish,</u> that is, spiritual nourishment. The heart and self had been distracted in their efforts to guard the spiritual nourishment for the heart. The heart had been preoccupied with other, higher goals and had forgotten the spiritual nourishment because of the constant, persistent demands of the animal self's desires to be met. The fish here also symbolizes the whale that swallowed the

Prophet Jonah. The idea of spiritual nourishment swal-
lowing Jonah is in the symbolic sense and not to be
understood literally. The spiritual nourishment was
what the heart and the self needed. The heart had commanded the self to carry the spiritual nourishment (faith
in God) with them and to care for it at the time they
established the firm intention to undertake their spiritual struggle.

Mysteriously the spiritual nourishment came back to
life and it took its way, burrowed a path for itself and
dove into the sea of the body, just as it had been before
beginning the struggle. It generated a spectacular, wide
passage. As a result of this wide opening, its path
through the waters became clearly marked and the sea
waves did not close in on it. [This is similar to the cross-
ing of the Red Sea whereby the path permitted Prophet
Moses and his people to cross while it drowned Pharaoh
and his army. That is, the path created by spiritual nourishment will only allow the believer to tread.]

At that junction, the heart became exhausted, weary
and extremely hungry for spiritual nourishment. Therat,
(it) remembered the spiritual nourishment although the
heart had not experienced weariness or hunger previous
to this moment in the spiritual struggle. Upon remembering the spiritual nourishment, the heart thought
about satisfying its needs. The heart asked the self for
the needed spiritual nourishment, saying, "Bring us our
food." This indicates that the heart is experiencing this
longing in the light of day where it is conscious of the
body and its needs as opposed to what the heart experienced in the womb where desires are dormant and spiritual nourishment is driven directly into the body
through the mother and without personal input or feeling the need for it.

The heart said, "Indeed we are exhausted by our
journey." That is the exhaustion and difficulties associated with giving birth. The self replied, "You see! When
we rested near the bedrock," or the breast to feed, "I for-

got the fish," the spiritual nourishment because it was not needed then. It was Satan, the one without hope, that made me forget by clouding my conscience. It is also narrated that the heart was resting when the spiritual nourishment came alive again and dove into the sea of the body. However, the self had been awake, guarding the heart when Satan caused the self to forget the spiritual nourishment. The self had been guarding the heart and the spiritual nourishment which was for the heart.

Even though the self had remained awake and vigilant in regard to the heart, it was made forgetful of the spiritual nourishment by Satan. In the same way that Satan had caused Adam to eat of the forbidden, so Satan caused the self to forget the spiritual nourishment. Spiritual nourishment then burrowed its path into the body. The self added, " so that I should not remember," that is, Satan made me forgetful of the spiritual nourishment. This is because the state of the self was distracted. The path mentioned in the story here symbolizes the condition of the body described earlier.

The heart had been asleep and forgot the spiritual nourishment because the heart had been overwhelmed, astonished, bewildered, shocked by its birth—"and so it took its way into the sea in a marvelous manner." What was amazing was the hole through which the spiritual nourishment passed. The spiritual nourishment escaped and made its own way which is the way of the animal self which naturally behaves like a youth who is rebellious and wants to make its own way by itself. It is in the nature of youth to try to escape and this is also the nature of the animal self.

The heart said, "This is what we were seeking!" This is the meeting that had been promised to the heart if it were turned towards spiritual nourishment, if it remembered its spiritual aspect. It is promised to the heart that it will meet something more knowledgeable than it, that is, the sacred intellect ('aql qudsi). Rising to

the state of perfection must be done through guidance
from the sacred intellect and this will only happen at
that junction where the two seas meet, and <u>so they
returned upon their tracks</u>, in returning to the state of
the nature originated by God (*fiṭrat Allāh*), the state in
which Adam had been created, a state they had been in
at an earlier stage [like Adam and Eve's original nature
before they did what they had been forbidden to do].
The heart, also, had forgotten, forgotten the spiritual
nourishment because it had been bewildered, amazed.
<u>Retracing</u> their steps, just as to narrate a story is to
retrace back to what happened otherwise it would not
be a story. A story goes back to a point and builds level
upon level. Descending, falling, they retraced their steps
in moving towards perfection and wisdom towards the
Real. They retraced back until they met the sacred intellect.

Then they found one of Our servants (Khidr) <u>unto
whom We had given mercy from Us</u>, who had been
given essential perfection, spiritual perfection by being
detached from the elements thereby attaining the spiritual, being above direction, absolute effulgence which is
the retracing of the story of being nigh unto God and in
His Presence, and <u>We had taught him knowledge</u>, spiritual knowledge (*'ilm ladūnnī*), which is knowledge <u>pro-
ceeding</u> directly <u>from Us</u>. That is, there is something
inside the human being which recognizes God and that
is His own knowledge from the sacred, Divine knowledge and absolute Truth, which came to him without
need of any human intermediary to teach and which is
not acquired through creation but only from what He
Himself expresses.

The heart <u>said to</u> (the sacred intellect)<u>, "May I follow
you so that you teach me of what you have been taught,
right judgment?"</u> that is, the manifestation of the will-
ingness to be of good conduct and to rise to that perfection. The sacred intellect said, <u>"Assuredly you will not
be able to bear with me patiently."</u> That is, you have no

knowledge of the hidden orders of the spiritual and the meaning behind spiritual truths. This is because you are not detached from the body and the senses. They veil you so that you will not be able to bear with me patiently. That is why it says, "How could you bear patiently that which you have never encompassed in your knowledge?" The heart said, "Yet you shall find me, if God will, patient " because I am prepared and I am persistent "and I shall not rebel against you in anything" because I came to you of my own accord and because I accepted you for my own moral healing. Your commands will benefit my own clarity and will prove the sincerity and truthfulness of my will. My intention is sincere. [The spiritual hermeneutic says: I speak to you with the tongue of the moment.] The sacred intellect said, "Then if you follow me, do not question me on anything until I myself introduce the mention of it to you." You must follow all the steps that I take. That is, you must follow my example, walk with determination and pursue the way with the performance of spiritual exercises to attain the best conduct and to struggle against your desires. Do not ask for any explanations of the inner truth. When the time is right, I will explain some of the hidden, spiritual meanings and truths to you. That is, "I will explain it to you when you become detached from your outer physical form and free from both the emotional influences of the heart and the senses."

So they departed until when they embarked upon a ship. That is, the body, mature enough, to perform the religious obligations. The sacred intellect took both the self and the heart and rode in the body. They went with the body to the sacred universe in the endless ocean to proceed towards God. The sacred intellect made a hole in the body, that is, it made the body defective through extra spiritual exercises and lessening of food intake so that the body could not go on its own, could no longer rebel. It was in a weakened state. He caused imperfection in its regular order. The heart said, "What, have you made a hole in it so as to drown its passengers?" That is, "Have you made it defective so as to break and weaken its animal and plant natures in this huge ocean so it will drown?" The heart said, "You have indeed done a grievous thing." This criticism shows that the heart is inclining towards the body because the heart is no longer able to fulfill the desires of the animal self and it is not content with the rights given to it. The sacred intellect said, "Did I not say that you could never bear with me patiently?" This is a spiritual challenge and a discipline showing that one's determination in conduct has to be stronger than that. The heart said, "Do not take me to task that I forgot, neither ask me to do a thing too difficult." That is, this is the station of the reproaching self (nafs al-lawwāmah).

So they departed until when they met a lad. This is the self in all its aspects which veils the heart and becomes the aspect of the self commanding to evil. The sacred intellect slew (it). It killed the aspect of the self which commands to evil and veils the heart by over-coming the faculties of avoidance of harm/pain (anger) and of the attraction to pleasure (desires).

The heart said, "What, have you slain an innocent soul and that not to retaliate for a soul slain?" That is, have you killed a soul that was innocent? The heart had compassion for the self and all its aspects. It is part of the nature of the heart to have compassion. "You have indeed done a horrible thing." The sacred intellect said, "Did I not say that you could never bear with me patiently?" Again, a spiritual challenge. The heart said, "If I question you on anything after this, then do not keep company with me. You have already experienced excuse sufficient on my part." The heart once again apologized and confessed to its wrongdoing and fail-ures. The reproaching aspect of self (nafs al-lawwāmah) has many forms, takes on many colors.

So they departed until when they reached the people

of a city, that is, the physical forces of the body, and they asked the people, the physical forces, for food, spiritual nourishment, but they refused. That is, they refused to give them spiritual nourishment, to receive them hospitably. The sacred intellect and the heart had been given spiritual nourishment from the sacred lights before their manifestation. Spiritual nourishment is a manifestation of Divine Beauty from above, knowledge from above. It cannot be given by the physical forces. Spiritual nourishment had come from the upper Light from where sacred knowledge and spiritual meanings come. This knowledge did not come before the body had been damaged and the aspect of the self commanding to evil had been killed through spiritual exercises. Before that time, the physical forces, the senses and feelings were a veil obstructing the heart and not a supplier of spiritual nourishment. While the body is occupied with doing spiritual exercises, it will cease interfering in the heart's ability to know God. Spiritual nourishment cannot be delivered until these forces are calm and quiet.

There they found a wall, that is, the self at peace (nafs al-muṭma'innah). The proof of this is that they found the wall after they had killed the self commanding to evil through spiritual exercises. The aspect of the self commanding to evil could not move by its own will. It had become motionless and because of its weakness, it had nearly died so the state of the aspect of the self at peace is described as the wall, exhausted and about to tumble down and so the sacred intellect set it up. It raised it up again through good conduct, behavior and attaining positive traits because of the manifestation of the light of the power of goodness. At that point, positive traits were able to rise above the negative. The heart said, "If you had wished, you could have taken a wage for that." This saying by the heart is from the animal self asking for immediate reward for doing good. The heart at this point is exhausted by the spiritual exercises. The sacred intellect said, "This is the parting between me and you," that is, between my station and your station and my state and your state.

In order to build up and strengthen the self at peace, spiritual exercises must be undertaken. This means not expecting a reward for manifesting praiseworthy conduct. Otherwise it is not a positive trait, not a praiseworthy deed and not a perfect deed. Attaining the positive traits is to manifest the Divine Qualities. That is praiseworthy. This emanates from a person who attains the positive traits in order to make a statement, to express something and not to get something out of it. God does not gain anything from creating us. It is this kind of deed that must be followed. Whatever one does for a reward acts as a veil and a wrongdoing. Trying to gain reward from it has a negative effect. The point is to drop the veil and expose the real quality of the nature of the soul at peace. God wants to expose them and only then can the soul at peace rise to the world of light to receive spiritual knowledge—the understanding of the meaning of things—to manifest the Divine Qualities.

"Now I will tell you the interpretation of that which you could not bear patiently." Now that the self is at peace and the physical forces have lost their strength, the heart is in a receptive state. It is prepared to receive knowledge of what it had earlier not been prepared to receive. The interpretation could only be explained when the heart is ready to accept meanings and inner knowledge. "As for the ship, it belonged to certain poor men who toiled upon the sea," that is, the physical forces which work for a living in the endless ocean of God. They are expressed by the outer senses and the natural plant forces. They are called poor because they are always silent and always attached to the body. They are weak and cannot oppose the heart and decide to go their own way dominating over the heart like other animal forces are capable of doing. They are similar to the limbs of the body and not like the faculties of the avoidance of harm/pain and the attraction to pleasure, the latter of which has a rebellious animal nature. It is said that the poor people were ten brothers. Five lived in time and five in the space of the endless ocean of the body. This indicates the inner and outer senses. They are weakened by spiritual exercises.

"I desired to damage [the ship] for behind them there was a king who was seizing every ship with brutal force." This king is the animal self (*nafs al-ammārah*) which will no longer be able to arise to seize them. This was the king who wanted to take over. The animal self was made defective so the king could not use the the body for its own lust and pleasure. As for the lad, his parents, the spirit and the body, were believers consenting and confessing to monotheism and submitting to the Divine Omnipotence willing, obeying and worshipping God. They were present whenever His call came "and we were afraid he would impose on them insolence and unbelief" and become a burden on them showing selfishness, ingratitude and disobedience to the spirit and the heart and not recognizing the good things they had done, thereby veiling them. The sacred intellect says, "We were afraid that the aspect of the self commanding to evil would spoil the faith of the spirit and heart and nullify the benefits of their worship." The spirit and the heart are created to do as God says.

" So we desired that their Lord should give to them in exchange one better than he in purity and nearer in tenderness," and that replacement was the soul at peace which is more sincere, purer, more merciful, more compassionate. The spirit and the heart have more compassion towards the self and the body and they are more useful to them.

As for the wall, it belonged to two orphan lads, theoretical and practical wisdom which were not connected to the Holy Spirit because of the influence and interference of the physical body. The body separated these two types of wisdom from their connection to the Holy

Spirit <u>in the city</u>, that is, <u>of</u> the body, and <u>under it was a</u> <u>treasure belonging to them</u>, that is, and beneath the soul at peace there was a treasure which is gnosis (*ma'rifah*) which can only be reached in the station of the heart because it is possible for the macrocosm and the microcosm to exist at the same time, at the time of perfection. That is the state of nearing higher realms, attaining what is most important. This is the time to extract the treasure. Some of the commentators of the outer meaning have said that the treasure was some scrolls that described who their parents were.

<u>Their father was a righteous man and your Lord</u> <u>desired that they should come of age and then bring</u> <u>forth their treasure as a mercy from your Lord.</u> This could also refer to their spiritual father who had been preserved for them and that is why this father is none other than the Holy Spirit. "<u>I did it not of my own bid-</u> <u>ding. This is the interpretation of that which you could</u> <u>not bear patiently</u>" (18:57-83).[1]

In the spiritual hermeneutics of this story, Moses symbolizes the heart in fluctuation between the body—physical desires— and the animal self—psychic demands. The latter is symbolized by the attendant or page to Moses who traditional commentators have said is Joshua. The place of the heart's encounter with the spiritual world is at the place in the body where the two seas—one sweet water and one salty—meet. This is the station of the heart. The fish symbolizes spiritual nourishment—faith in the One God at the deepest level. When the heart remembers its spiritual nourishment, it asks the self—the cognitive psychic forces within—perception and motivation—to bring it. The self is amazed that it has lost the spiritual nourishment saying that Satan, that which has no hope, caused it to forget so it would not be able to remember. The heart realizes this is what it had been promised so the heart retraces its steps along with the self back to its nature

originated by God (*fiṭrat Allāh*). With the Light of the
nature originated by God, the heart is then given a meeting with the sacred intellect. While traditional commentators say that the one with whom Moses is promised a
meeting, with someone who is more knowledgeable than
he is, is Khidr, the "Green Man," the inner guide who
comes to a person in their dreams, is symbolized by the
sacred intellect. The sacred intellect is that aspect of nature
to which God gives knowledge of Himself directly.

The heart asks to accompany the sacred intellect and
although the sacred intellect doubts the heart's preparedness or receptivity to bear patiently the things that it
encounters, it agrees when the heart reassures the sacred
intellect of its commitment and strength of will.

Three circumstances are encountered: a ship, symbolized by the body of the spiritual warrior, which the sacred
intellect damages through strenuous spiritual exercises
like superogatory prayers, extra fasting and "remembering
God" (*dhikr*) sessions.

Secondly, they encounter a lad symbolized as that
aspect of self which commands to the negative as opposed
to commanding to the positive and preventing the development of the negative. The sacred intellect kills that
aspect of self which commands to the negative because it
is effecting the faith in the One God of the inner spirit and
the body, symbolized by the lad's parents. Finally, they
come to a wall which is crumbling. The wall symbolizes
the self at peace, the stage when once attained is described
as tranquility by the spiritual warrior.

At each of the encounters, the heart questions the
sacred intellect. In other words, it has not as yet detached
itself from the body and the outer senses. It still turns
towards compassion for them. It is only after the body
(ship) is weakened through strenuous spiritual exercises,
after the aspects of the self that command to the negative
(the lad) is killed and after the self at peace (the crumbling

wall) is rebuilt, revived, that the heart is able to accept the inner interpretation, the spiritual meaning of what the sacred intellect had done.

At each encounter, the heart comments to the sacred intellect about what had taken place. When it is challenged in a spiritual way by the sacred intellect for its interference and comments, which is other than to bear patiently with the sacred intellect, the heart reproaches itself for having questioned the acts of the sacred intellect. This is symbolized as the appearance of the reproachful self (*nafs lawāmmah*).

In terms of psychoethics, Moses symbolizes the heart located in the center of self. Through the struggles in which it engages, it becomes morally healed, balanced in justice (putting Reality in Its proper place) which is symbolized by the self at peace (*nafs muṭma'innah*). The heart attains this stage by first returning to its nature originated by God (*fiṭrat Allāh*), retracing its steps back to where it has been promised a meeting with something more knowledgeable than the heart is. It must begin by decreasing the influence of physical and psychic desires and demands. This is accomplished through strenuous spiritual exercises like superogatory prayers, extra fasting and "remembrance of God" (*dhikr*) sessions (putting a hole in the ship). Once the body is weakened, the animal aspects of self are also weakened.

The animal aspects of self are referred to as the *nafs ammārah*. This consists of two functions: avoidance of harm/pain and attraction to pleasure. They are known collectively as the passions (feelings and actions). They are symbolized by the lad in the story. When the aspect of the self which commands to the negative or the animal aspect of self is slain, the heart can then manifest courage (trust in the One God) and temperance (charity towards others).

Each time the heart confronts the sacred intellect for its actions, the heart reproaches itself for not having borne the experience patiently. This symbolizes the appearance of the reproaching aspects of self (*nafs lawāmmah*, reason) or theoretical and practical wisdom (belief in the One God and practice of the Law and the Way).

DHUL QARNAYN

They ask you (Muhammad) concerning Dhul Qarnayn. Say: I will recite to you a mention of him. We have established him in the land and have granted him means to everything and he followed a way until when he reached the setting of the sun. He found it setting in a spring of boiling water and there he found a community.

We said: Oh Dhul Qarnayn, as for the wrongdoer, we shall chastise him then when he is returned to his Lord. He will subject him to a shastisement beyond description. But as for him who believes and does righteous work, there is the most excellent reward and we shall speak to him mild commands.

Then he followed a Way until the rising of the sun. He found it rising upon a community for whom We had provided no covering to protect them from it. He did the same with them and We certainly encompassed in knowledge all about him.

Then he followed a Way until he approached two dams. He found in front of them a community hardly able to understand speech. They said: Oh Dhul Qarnayn, Gog and Magog are indeed corrupting the earth so shall we assign a tribute to you in order that you may set up a barrier between us and them? He said: What my Lord has established me in is better. So you help me vigorously and I will set up a rampart between you and them. Bring me ingots of iron until when he had made all level between the two cliffs. He said, 'Blow,' until when he made it a fire. He said, "Bring me molten brass to pour thereon.' Thus they were unable to surmount it nor were they ever able to tunnel through it. But when my Lord's promise comes to pass, He will level it to the earth and my Lord's promise is ever the Truth (18:84-98).

The spiritual hermeneutics follow:

They ask you (Muhammad) concerning Dhul Qarnayn. They say he was from the Eastern Roman Empire and lived not long ago. In terms of practice, Dhul Qarnayn refers to the heart which has two horns, two wings, the East and the West. Say: 'I will recite to you a mention of him.' We have established him in the land and have granted him means to everything. We gave him strength in the land and power over the body. The heart had power over the body. This story differs from the above story of Moses for here the heart is the king whose power reaches everywhere. God gave the heart power and it was capable of earning any wealth it wanted in the macrocosm or the microcosm and to walk wherever it wanted. It was given perfection in every way in order to reach its goals. and (it) followed a way that responded to the body until when (it) reached the setting of the sun. This is where the spirit sets. He found it setting in a spring of boiling water, that is, like hot springs, the state of the body when it is digesting food and there he found a community. That is, the forces of the self, the body, the senses, the spiritual forces and the inspirational forces.

We said: 'Oh Dhul Qarnayn,' oh heart, you could either chastise them through spiritual exercises and killing them practically or adopt a way of kindness towards them and adopt a middle way and give each their share of what they need. It said, 'As for the wrong-doer,' by indulging in excess and not following the rules and following lust, desires, anger, illusions and allusions, 'we shall chastise them' with spiritual exercises and 'then when he is returned to his Lord,' that is, at the time of death, 'He will subject him to a chastisement beyond description.' He will cast them into the fire of nature where they will be tormented. This is more difficult to bear than the punishment on the Day of Resurrection. They will be annihilated. 'But as for him who believes' through cognizance and practical and theoretical wisdom, who admonish the senses to attain the positive traits, an exalted state, 'and does righteous work' through submission, 'there is the most excellent reward' of the paradise of the attributes and manifestation of His lights. There will be light from their faces and flowing of rivers of knowledge by which you will recognize the believer. They will face the light when it separates from the profusion of knowledge, 'and we shall speak to him mild commands'.

Then (it) followed a Way until it reached the path that leads to God by renouncing any material attachment, seeking higher ground, the rising of the sun, that is, where the spirit rises. (It) found it rising upon a community who are two wise ones: theoretical and practical wisdom and spiritual strength for whom We had provided no covering to protect them from it because they are light and because they understand fully the spiritual meaning as described earlier. He did the same with them and We certainly encompassed in knowledge all about him. They had acquired the perfections of the exalted attributes. No one but Us knows about this because God is Omnipresent in both universes at the same time. No one in the universe can have such perfect knowledge except God and because of what is known as the Throne of God.

Then (it) followed a Way until (it) approached two dams, meaning the two universes and that is his state and original station walking between the East and the West. This is a journey that sits it in its rightful position in exaltation. (It) found in front of them a community, a community of human beings, physical forces and outer senses, hardly able to understand speech because the physical forces and outer senses do not know words and cannot speak. They said with the tongue of the present: 'Oh Dhul Qarnayn, Gog', that is, claims, suspicion, idiosity, supersensitiveness 'and Magog', imagination and superstition, 'are indeed corrupting the earth' of the body. They entice the body to indulge in their desires and to seek pleasures that are against what is orderly in the universe and encourage them to do deeds that bring imbalances and hinder the laws of attaining the positive traits like wisdom. They cause corruption in the body and desires, lust and innovation which are against justice and which lead to the corruption of the seeds of the next generation.

They were denigrated so they said to the heart, 'Shall we assign a tribute,' some of our strength 'to you in order that you may set up a barrier between us and them?' so that we may overcome desires by setting up a barrier between our hearts and them that will manifest as practical wisdom. (It) said, 'What my Lord has established me in is better (than your tribute),' meaning that what God gave me the meanings which result from practical experience, the knowledge of the macrocosm and the microcosm and the ability to travel with ease from the East to the West, to attain positive traits and follow God's commands which God created you to do 'so you help me vigorously and I will set up a rampart between you and them.' That dam is practical wisdom and the Shariah.

(It) said, 'Bring me ingots of iron,' from the practical images and do what you are ordered to do with firmness and certitude, Until when he had made all level between the two cliffs, by balancing and by measuring the correct needs of both sides. Then it said to the animal forces, 'Blow,' life into the microcosm so its meaning becomes more significant and blow on the varying psychological manifestations including good qualities, blow until when he made it a fire, that is, knowledge as part of universal knowledge while practical knowledge is particular knowledge of what to do.

(It) said, 'Bring me molten brass to pour thereon,' that is, the intention and sense of purpose which must exist between knowledge and actions. Knowledge without intentions and actions without purpose are not rewarded. With that molten lead, the spirit of knowledge will become one—not divided—and with it the spirit of knowledge and the body of actions will become one and united by molten lead. This is similar to the animal self standing between the human self and the body. There was a barrier there, a veil, a foundation, a structure based on deeds and this was knowledge, conduct and the lead of intention and purpose. Then the self became the self at peace and recognized its original nature (*fiṭrat Allāh*) and felt comfort and peace, understanding its intended state and believed.

Thus they were unable to surmount it nor were they ever able to tunnel through it because it was exalted and because it contained all kinds of knowledge and proof which could neither be rejected nor overcome. The body and the senses are too ignorant of the truth to overcome it and to pierce through it. They took control of all the capabilities. This barrier is the Divine Law, the Shariah. He said: The Divine Law is a mercy from my Lord to servants which brings them peacefulness, tranquillity and maintains them. 'But when my Lord's promise comes to pass,' that is, when death comes, 'He will level ' the body 'to the earth' because it does not work when it is dead, without the soul or spirit 'and my Lord's promise is ever the Truth.' [2]

In this story, the role of the heart (Dhul Qarnayn) differs from its role in the story of Moses and Khidr above. Here we are told the heart is king whose power reaches everywhere. This story symbolizes the heart as the Throne of God based on the Divine Tradition, "My heavens and My earth do not embrace Me but the heart of My believing servant embraces Me."

The heart first encounters the place where the spirit sets. This place is within the body when it is occupied with absorbing food. We also learn that the body consists of "a community" of forces which include along with itself, sensible, psychic and spiritual forces. As long as these forces obey the king—the heart—the self at peace—they can be contained through spiritual exercises or adopting a "middle way," a way of moderation towards them. But whatever sensible, psychic or spiritual forces that follow the way of excess, they are the wrongdoers. This excess may come in the form of lust, desires, anger, illusions or allusions. Whatever it may be, if it takes the heart, the king, the self at peace away from moral balance and harmony, it is to be chastised with spiritual exercises just as those aspects of self which believe will be rewarded.

The heart next traveled to the place where the spirit rises. It rises upon wisdom, both practical and theoretical. They had no covering over the spirit because they are also made of light.

Two dams are then approached by the heart—the East and the West. The community there—physical forces— complained of aspects of self which were corrupting the body with their suspiciousness and superstitiousness. They cause moral imbalance. They oppose wisdom and justice and corrupt the next generation as well.

The community wanted to strengthen the heart but the heart declined their offer saying God had already given it understanding of the inner meaning of practical knowl- edge—like the crafts—along with knowledge of the macrocosm and the microcosm—spiritual astrology and spiritual alchemy. The heart has also been given the ability to travel with ease between the East and the West and to attain the positive traits of courage, temperance, wisdom and justice.

Using the practical wisdom of a craftsman, the heart is able to set up a barrier between suspicion and superstition and the community of physical forces. The barrier the heart built to keep them out is practical wisdom and the Law. The heart leveled the earth of the body between the two dams and built a barrier of the Law to keep out nega- tive thoughts. Everything was measured and held in bal- ance. The heart then told the animal aspects of self to bring it iron or practical knowledge and then to blow life, the spirit, breath into the microcosm of the self so that its meaning grow in significance. It is told to blow until it cre- ates a fire, universal knowledge, which melts even iron. Molten brass, symbolizing one's good intention, is used to connect one's knowledge and actions because an act done or knowledge attained without first intending to do it for God's sake is not rewarded.

CHAPTER 4: SPIRITUAL STAGES

Spiritual chivalry is traditionally viewed as movement through three stages: moral goodness (*murūwwah*), spiritual chivalry in its particular sense (*futuwwah*), and sanctity or the stage of the friend of God (*walāyah*).

MORAL GOODNESS

Depending upon the century and where the spiritual warrior lived, he or she might have had access to traditional centers of learning where the manifest sciences like that of ethics would be taught. If the spiritual warrior lived in an era of decline of traditional centers of learning, he or she might have found a Sufi center where the hidden sciences would be taught, namely, the sciences of numbers, geometry, letters and spiritual alchemy and spiritual astrology.

Centers like these are less available for the 20th century aspiring spiritual warrior but God has not left them without recourse to at least be able to heal morally through a self-help method based in the practice of self-examination. Without a master and a group, even greater motivation and will is required to endure the perils of the struggle at this first stage. No one but God knows how many have tried and given up but those that have succeeded in either consciously or unconsciously attaining the stage of moral goodness are apparent by observing how they relate to God and God's people—their husband, wife, child, children, family, neighbor, co-worker, teachers and so forth. They are people who have not only experienced the Divine Signs within and without but have first read them, become conscious of them, and then proceeded to experience them.

The first stage a master puts his or her disciple through is that of *murūwwah*. Without the presence of a master, this first stage is possible to attain using the Sign of

53

the Presence of God as originally developed by the Naqshbandi Sufis in Central Asia (a form of what in the West is called the Enneagram). This can be an invaluable aid to the aspiring spiritual warrior at this stage of moral development as will be explained, whether or not he or she be under the direction of a master. Using the method presented here, which developed through centuries of oral tradition and personal experiences of pious people, the spiritual warrior engages self in combat seeking to influence the heart to turn towards the spiritual and away from the desires and demands of the idol/ego within.

If the spiritual warrior has a master, he or she would most likely be part of a group and this group participation further enhances moral development as it is preceeded by an initiation ceremony which symbolically connects the spiritual warrior to the Source. This is what is referred to as the second stage (*futuwwah*) while joining a group may in actuality even precede the stage of moral goodness (*murūwwah*). Whatever the circumstances, moral healing precedes spiritual development.

Murūwwah literally means "manliness." Even though it may sound to be a gender specific term, it has never traditionally been interpreted as such although historically far more men have manifested this model than women. There are many factors behind this historical fact, a discussion of which would take us far beyond the scope of this work. Suffice it to say that the term is not interpreted as being gender specific as evidenced by the words of Ibn al-'Arabī, the great Muslim mystic. When he refers to a group of friends of God, he says, "Everything we mention about these men by the term 'men' may include women, although most often men are mentioned." One of the friends of God asked, "How many are they?" He answered, "Forty souls." He was asked, "Why do you not say forty men?" He answered, "Because there may be women among them."[1] About a woman Sufi Ibn al-'Arabī remarks, "I have never seen one more chivalrous than her in our time."[2]

Many positive traits are associated with "manliness" which either gender may attain. It is not gender which assures success but commitment and perseverance in rigorous, constant self-examination. It is to keep reason as an aspect of the spirit alive and active while preparing the animal aspects of self (the passions) to be receptive of Divine Grace.

A full definition of *murūwwah* is

> ....to abstain from things unlawful; to be temperant in manners and to have some trade or craft; to abstain from doing secretly what one would be ashamed to do openly; or to be in the habit of doing what is approved, and shunning what is held base; or in preserving the soul from reprehensible actions and what disgraces in the estimation of people; or good manners and guarding the tongue and shunning impudence; or a quality of the mind, the preserving of which makes a person persevere in good manners and habits... In a word, it is virtue; or rather manly virtue or moral goodness.[3]

To attain moral goodness is to become a morally reasonable, religiously cultured monotheist (*ḥalīm*). This is the goal of the spiritual warrior at the stage of *murūwwah*. In order to attain this goal, the spiritual warrior develops the traits which describe a monotheist (*ḥanīf*), one who submits to God's Will (*muslim*), one who is a servant (*'abd*) of God and one who is a believer (*mu'min*). It is then that the spiritual warrior manifests *ḥilm*, the moral reasonableness of a religiously cultured monotheist.

MONOTHEIST

As a monotheist (*ḥanīf*), the spiritual warrior is in touch with his or her nature originated by God (*fiṭrat Allāh*) and follows the example of Prophet Abraham.

"Abraham, a monotheist..." (4:125) and *"follow the creed of Abraham, a monotheist..."* (3:95). Abraham was *"a monotheist and no idolater"* (16:120).

SUBMISSIVE TO GOD'S WILL

Prophet Abraham was not only a model as a monotheist but as one submissive to God's Will, as well. *"(Abraham) was one who submitted to God's Will (muslim) and a monotheist..."* (3:67). This is also referred to in the Quran as the natural religion of mankind which is part of human nature originated by God (30:30). Even as a community the Quran councils people to only worship God as monotheists, *"and to perform the ritual prayer and to give in charity. This is the true (community)"* (98:5). For spiritual warriors, using the founder of spiritual chivalry, Prophet Abraham, as a model, the Sign in the Quran is telling them not to associate anything with God.

This is a step taken by spiritual warriors as their existential position in moving towards their Lord. A Sign in the Quran of the prayer of Abraham and Ishmael after rebuilding the Kabah confirms this view of the spiritual warrior: *"Our Lord, make us submissive (muslim) to You and of our seed a nation submissive..."* (2:128). The religion of Prophet Abraham is specifically referred to in the Sign that says,

> When his Lord said to him, 'Submit,' and he said, 'I submit to the Lord of all Being.' And this was the legacy that Abraham left to his sons and Jacob likewise: 'My sons, God has chosen for you the religion. See that you die not except in submission (to His Will)' (2:131-132).

The spiritual warrior recites,

> And struggle for God as is His due for He has chosen you and imposed no difficulties on you in religion being the creed of your father Abraham. He named you 'those who submit to the Will of God (muslim)' (22:78)

SERVANT OF THE LORD

The servant of the Lord follows the model of Prophet Muhammad who is referred to in the Quran as God's servant[4] as are Joseph,[5] David[6] and Job,[7] Moses and Aaron,[8] and Elias.[9]

The Quran says, *"God is never unjust to His servants..."* (3:182). Iblis has no authority over God's servant.[10] It is to the servant that God sends clear Signs *"...that He may lead you from the depths of darkness into the Light..."* (57:9).

When My servants ask you concerning Me, I am indeed close (to them): I listen to the prayer of every supplicant when he calls on Me. Let them also, with a will, listen to My Call and believe in Me that they may walk in the right way (2:186). God is gentle with His servants... (2:207). Say to My servants that they should (only) say those things that are best ... (17:53).

The servants of the Merciful are those who walk on the earth in humility and when the ignorant address them, they say, 'Peace'. Those who spend the night in worship of their Lord, prostrate and standing... (25:63-64).

Those who when they spend are not extravagant and not niggardly but hold a just (balance) between those (extremes). Those who invoke not with God any other god nor slay such life as God has made sacred except for just cause, nor commit fornication...and who repent and do good have truly turned to God with a conversion. Those who witness no falsehood and, if they pass by futility, they pass by it with honorable (avoidance) (25:67-72).

And they are told,

My servants! No fear shall be on you that Day nor shall you grieve—being those who have believed in Our Signs and submitted (to God's Will) (43:69).

Believer

According to the Quranic description, spiritual warriors attaining the last level of the stage of moral goodness, the moral reasonableness of a religiously cultured monotheist, constantly perform devotional exercises. They fear the Day of Judgment, do acts of charity without being either ostentatious or boastful about it, distances self from acts done out of ignorance of Reality which God has forbidden like worshipping other than the One God, slaying a living being without right, and so forth.

> *Believers are those who when God is mentioned feel a tremor in their hearts and when they hear His Signs rehearsed, find their faith strengthened and put (all) their trust in their Lord; Who establish regular prayers and spend (freely) out of the gifts We have given them for sustenance. Such in truth are the believers. They have grades of dignity with their Lord and forgiveness and generous sustenance (8:2-4). It is not fitting for a believer, man or woman, when a matter has been decided by God and His Messenger, to have any option about their decision. If anyone disobeys God and His Messenger, he is indeed on a clearly wrong path (33:36). Believers are but a single brotherhood... (49:10).*

True faith requires action and action for the sake of God is the very substance of the spiritual warrior.

Morally Healed: Manifesting Moral Goodness and Reasonableness

Positive traits (virtues) are the fruits of Divine Grace. They are infused as potential within the human being at the time of the infusion of the Divine Spirit and in this sense they are gifts of God. On the other hand, they also have to be actualized by the human being in his struggle and striving against the idol within in order to become worthy of the gifts.

The Quran refers to believers saying,

> *The true believers are those who believe in God and His Messenger and afterwards never doubt (who have wisdom), but struggle (in God's Cause) with their wealth (having temperance) and with their lives (having courage) in the Way of God. These are the truthful ones (being just).* (49:15).

Moral goodness is symbolized for the spiritual warrior through four basic positive traits as has been mentioned. They are courage, wisdom, temperance and justice. The first three have multiple sub-categories while the fourth means attaining balance and centeredness thereby unveiling the spiritual qualities of the heart.

WISDOM

The pillars of *murūwwah* are three things in terms of wisdom are of which point the spiritual warrior to faith in the One God:

> First, to live with oneself by intellect, to live with creatures in patience, to live with God through need. To live with oneself by intellect is to know the measure of oneself, to see the dimension of one's work, to strive for one's own good. To live with creatures in patience is being satisfied with them when they are strong, seeking out excuses for them and deciding in their favor when you are strong. To live with God through need is to give thanks for whatever comes from Him, to forget what one did for Him and to see His choice as correct.[11]

Wisdom for the spiritual warrior is from the positive trait from which all others develop. Wisdom as faith in the One God is based on knowledge of God which God Himself has given through the nature originated by Him (*fiṭrat Allāh*). As spiritual warriors come to know self they see God's providence in regard to all creatures, His care in providing them with sustenance and His protection of them. This knowledge for spiritual warriors is confirmed and made clear by the Quran and *sunnah*.

Wisdom in the sense of faith in God opposes disbelief and ingratitude (*kufr*). Morally healed spiritual warriors are concerned *"with doing pious deeds in this world while the unbeliever seeks after worldly pleasures"* (47:12). While spiritual warriors fight in the cause of God, disbelievers fight for the cause of idols, the ego which spiritual warriors have eliminated through the struggle. Spiritual warriors manifesting wisdom through their faith as monotheists, submitters to God's Will, servants of God and believers read the Sign, *"...there is no compulsion in religion..."* (2:256) from their position of moral reasonableness. They know their Lord has the power to compel people to believe but does not do so. The Lord is rather Merciful, Compassionate and Forgiving. As trustees of nature, they manifest the behavioral patterns of their Lord rather than those of their own idol/ego within.

According to spiritual chivalry, wisdom consists of both faith and actions, wisdom itself often being divided between the theoretical and practical—faith and good deeds. While having faith is considered a deed by itself, here the deed results from God's guidance. Hujwīrī says, "Faith is really the act of the human being joined to the guidance of God. Inclination to believe is the guidance of God while belief is the act of the human being."[12]

God's inclination towards the spiritual warrior results in a conviction about Reality as a possible human response. This conviction, in turn, empowers the spiritual warrior to direct his or her will to doing good deeds in submission to a higher Will. The stronger the inclination to believe, the less room for doubt. *"He gives wisdom to whomsover He will and whoso is given wisdom has been given much good..."* (2:269). *"True believers are those who believe in God and His Messenger and afterwards never doubt..."* (49:15).

COURAGE

Courage in terms of moral goodness (*murūwwah*) has three signs and for the spiritual warrior means trust in God:

Self-examination is to learn what your own moral imbalances are, to be grateful to God that your moral imbalances have been covered over and never to cease to fear God.[13] Spiritual chivalry manifested in its aspects of courage through socioethics is not to blame others for a defect that you know comes from yourself. It also has three Signs: "Never entertain suspicion in regard to things you do not know about them; cover over and hide what you do know; and become an intercessor, [at least in this world] for believers."[14]

It is based on a firm belief in God and the Last Day and in this sense, courage has direction. It is not a blind impulse as is ignorance of Reality but a noble, well-disciplined empowerment of the self with the goal of serving God's cause, *"striving (in God's cause) with your life"* (49:15).

It develops out of putting one's trust in God. An early Sufi notes,

Rely on Him, my brother, with the reliance of one who thinks rightly of Him, who has confidence in His promises and relies upon His fulfillment of them, whose heart has rest from anxiety because he trusts His words.[15]

It is through the development of a sense of trust that spiritual warriors then surrender self and all of the self's concerns into God's Hands. It is this that brings the spiritual warrior close to their Lord. With this, they lose concern for this world; no longer fear other than God; and no longer desire what others possess. The passions can no longer attract the heart away from its spiritual role. Tranquility and peace of mind follow because the self has given up all sense of anxiety about what might happen tomorrow and from where one's provisions will come. He will provide.

Al-Muḥāsibī explains this sense of trust which leads to courage for the spiritual warrior who "...*strives (for God's cause) with his life...*" (49:14).

> This trust means confiding to God all one's fears and hopes, placing no reliance on one's own strength and power or on that of the creatures, only on that of God, looking for no kindness or favor except from Him. The servant of God realizes that he has no control nor strength nor power nor dominion of his own which he needs to commit unto his Lord, for his Lord is overruling him and all his affairs. It means only that he willingly entrusts to his Lord that which He already controls and says within himself that he will commit his affairs to his Lord, Who controls all things. He attains to this state of trust through reflection and recollection and it means the cessation of all worldly anxieties and of hope and fear in regard to any creature for he knows that his Lord will supply his needs and, remembering that all things are in His hand, he seeks no help from any creature for his is the expectation of one who looks to his Lord and to no other. So trust follows upon dependence and dependence upon reliance. Because he depended upon Him, he trusted Him and committed to Him all his affairs, knowing that by Him all things are ordered aright.[16]

TEMPERANCE

Temperance means liberality and charity. With *ḥilm* it is not to show off, not to be wasteful, to keep to moderation.[17]

> *The parable of those who spend their sustenance in the Way of God is that of a grain of corn. It grows seven ears and each ear has a hundred grains. God gives manifold increase to*

whom He pleases and God cares for all... (2:261).

The giving of what one has, the sharing, the compassion and service to others fosters the positive trait of temperance when acting out of a sense of moral reasonableness. The negative side is to be stingy or miserly.

Al-Muḥāsibī says,

> It is required of you that you should seek good for others and not refuse it to them and that you should not desire evil for them. Do you fall short of this and are you content that people should desire good for you while you seek evil for them? And it is required of you that you should not set yourself above others, whether (inwardly) in your heart or (outwardly) by your tongue and it is required, too, that none should claim what is due from you to him and be refused.[18]

Al-Muḥāsibī summarizes the requirements of the virtue of charity in the Golden Rule, "Desire for others what you desire for yourself and avoid for them what you avoid for yourself."[19]

The spiritual warrior disciplines self in concealing gifts given to others. The Messenger said in this regard,

> When God created the earth and provided it with its inhabitants and created the mountains and established them that they should not be moved and laid the foundations of the earth, the angels said, 'God has created nothing stronger than the mountains.' Then God created iron and it cleft the mountains; then He created fire and behold it cleft the iron; and God commanded the water and it extinguished the fire; and He gave command to the wind and it stilled the water. And the angels were of different opinions about this and said, 'Oh Lord, which is the strongest of Your creatures which You have created?' and He said, 'I have created

nothing stronger than the son of Adam when he gives alms with his right hand and conceals it from his left hand and this is the strongest creature I have created.'[20]

JUSTICE

Justice, al-Muḥāsībī says, is of two kinds, outward justice between the servant and his fellow-servants and inward between the servant and his Lord. The road of justice is the direct road, along which it is obligatory for a man to travel. The just are characterized by knowledge of what is their duty, by action in accordance with that knowledge and by patience.

> The key to justice and the beginning of it for the servant is that he should know the worth of the self. It should have no worth in his eyes beyond its proper place and his inward self should correspond to its outward conduct. If there is that within him of which he would be ashamed if men could see it, it is for him to change his state to one of which he is not ashamed. The man who is farthest from justice is the one who is most neglectful of what is due to God and the one least given to self-examination.[21]

A sign of being a fair and just person according to Sufis is that you not have two rules in life, one for yourself and one for others but one single principle for both. Justice is to manifest a sense of order and discernment and it is defined by Hujwīrī as "putting everything in its proper place."[22] It is to be a person who reflects and perceives what is right by the light of his knowledge.

Spiritual warriors who have attained a sense of justice are described by al-Muḥāsībī:

> ....they oppose their own desires, fight against their enemy (without and within the self), put things in their right place through their knowledge and see to it that

affairs pursue their proper course. Thereby they realize what is due to God and its causes, occasions and occurrences and aspects in what these consist and what is to be put first, in accordance with God's law for the universe, including the human being. The first thing which is due to God and which justice requires should be rendered to Him, is worship and then right action in accordance with the observance of His law. It is with the due observance of the rights of God, on the part of the servant, that the servant serves the Lord as a matter of right and justice between them.[23]

Spiritual warriors are told, "The root is that the servant strive constantly for the sake of others. It is not to see self as superior to others. It is to act justly without demanding justice for yourself."[24] The Quran says, *"Be those who stand firmly in justice"* (4:135).

PIETY

Closely linked with justice for the spiritual warrior is piety (*taqwā*). It is defined by Talq b. Ḥabīb, a source used by al-Muḥāsibī, who said,

Piety is action in obedience to God, according to the Light received from God, in the hope of receiving His reward; it is the abandonment of disobedience to God, in accordance with the Light received from Him, in fear of His chastisement. True piety as regards the outward conduct is abiding in truth and abandoning disobedience and true piety as regards the inner life is the desire to fulfill all religious duties as unto God alone, in lowliness, with weeping and sorrow and prayer and fasting and all the acts of devotion to which God invites His servants without making them obligatory because of His loving-kindness and tender mercy towards them and what He invites them to is not found acceptable except through piety by which the desire therein is directed solely towards Him.[25]

Piety, like other positive traits, is derived from faith in the oneness of God and hence its direction towards serving Him alone. It is to avoid wrongdoing which is contrary to the One Will which controls the universe.

SPIRITUAL CHIVALRY

Spiritual chivalry (*futuwwah*) refers to both the second stage that spiritual warriors pass through as well as to the traditional craft guilds, athletics, neighborhood watch, military establishments, architects or artisan groups to which they may be attached through the presence of a spiritual master. While many women throughout Islamic history have gone through the stage of spiritual chivalry and moved towards the last stage, sanctity as a friend of God, very few have formed sisterhoods in areas where their male counterparts have. In other words, they may have had informal groups or been part of the brotherhoods, which did not exclude them, but rarely did they form their own spiritual organizations of craft guilds or artisans or athletics.

The spiritual warrior is described as one who "has no enemy, who honors those senior to him, who shows mercy to those junior or inferior to him, and prefers those who are his equals to himself."[26] It is to be "an enemy of your own idol/ego for the sake of your Lord."[27] The Sufi ideal of *ithār*, to give to others what you yourself need, is brought to its perfection in the *futuwwah* concept. The *fatā* is he who has no enemy and who does not care whether he is with a saint or an infidel.[28] The Messenger Muhammad was the perfect spiritual warrior for on the Day of Judgment, everybody will say "I" but he will say "My community."[29]

Very often spiritual warriors formed centers around a spiritual master where service to one another became the basis of the moral code. In a famous book for new aspirants to the Way, the master writes,

To render service to one's brethren is more valuable for the new aspirant than to be engaged in supererogatory prayers. Aiesha, the wife of the Prophet, said that the Prophet had always been busy with some charitable work.[30]

It is at the stage of spiritual chivalry in its group context that one undergoes a spiritual initiation. The spiritual warrior may be initiated and then begin the stages of *murūwwah* as pointed out earlier.

The initiation ceremony for the spiritual warrior traditionally involves three things which symbolize four positive traits. The first is the drinking of water and salt. Water symbolizes **wisdom** (faith in the One God) while salt symbolizes **justice** (putting Reality in Its proper place). The second is the wearing a pair of trousers or long pants. This is a symbol of **temperance** (charity, giving to others). The final act is the wearing of a belt which symbolizes **courage** (trust in God). These are the four positive traits that the spiritual warrior seeks to attain by returning to the nature originated by God.

The Nimatullahi Order particularly emphasizes service within the Sufi house itself.

The service is performed according to an ancient and well-defined code of behavior (*adab*) for as it is sometimes said, 'the whole of Sufism is *adab*.' The attitude of the Sufi in this service is one of altruistic purity (*ṣafā*) [moral healing] so that in interactions with others, each Sufi considers himself below the other. Furthermore, the Sufis are generally encouraged to seek proximity to God, the Creator through service to His creatures in society. According to the dictum, 'Selfhood is blasphe-my even if it be holy,' the Sufis' service has worth only to the degree that it is selfless and altruistic. Insofar as selfishness and egocentricity are the natural enemies of all spirituality, from the unitarian standpoint of the Nimatullahi Sufis, giving offense to a person is an offense against the Creator, whereas feeling offended by a creature is tantamount to maintaining an attitude of multitheism before the One Creator.[31]

FRIEND OF GOD

The last stage is *walāyah* (sanctity, the friend of God). Abraham was the first to move through the stages. The *walīs* are known as the ¨friends of God, as a person who takes God as a friend as the Quran says, *"My Friend is God...He befriends the just"* (7:196).

CHAPTER 5: SPIRITUAL PRACTICES

For various reasons throughout history, in the view of spiritual chivalry, while some people remained monotheists, having illuminated the inner Light of their nature originated by God, many began worshipping more gods than there were. This led to developments like the Greek or Hindu pantheon. The worship of other than the One God is considered to be a state of ignorance about Reality. It was for this reason that God sent Reminders and Reminderers to confirm the message of monotheism.

The spiritual warrior, through spiritual practices, moves out of the state of mystical participation with nature, separates from it by becoming consciously aware of his or her own existence, and gains knowledge of self following the Tradition, "He who knows himself, knows his Lord." Through the guidance of Reminders like the Quran, the spiritual warrior is led to knowledge of the self and Lord.

The most important practice of the spiritual warrior at the stage of developing *murūwwah*, moral goodness, is that of self-examination for it leads to moral healing and can be a self-help method if used in conjunction with the Sign of "the Presence of God." While traditionally the methods of spiritual chivalry are passed through oral tradition from one master to the next, there are similarities and differences among the methods but self-examination is an essential practice in all orders of spiritual chivalry. It is emphasized over and over again by the masters and is an important way of awakening the heart of the spiritual warrior to its spiritual aspects, moving on the way towards moral goodness.

Self-examination begins by knowing self. Algazel put it in the clearest prose when he said:

Know that the key to knowing God is knowing 'self'.
If you do not know your self, how will you know others? Moreover you may think that you know your self
and be mistaken for this kind of knowing is not the key
to the knowledge of Reality. The beasts know this much
of themselves. If you only know your outward head,
face, hands, feet, flesh and know that when you are hungry, you eat bread and when you are angry, you fall on
the other person and when attraction to pleasure dominates, you make for the marriage act, all the beasts
know that much. Therefore, you must seek your own
reality. From where have you come? Where will you go?
For what work have you come to this dwelling place?
Why were you created? If you want to know your 'self'
you should know that when you were created, two
things were created: one is the outward frame which is
called the body. It can be seen with the outward eye.
The second is the inward meaning which is called the
self, the spirit, and the heart. It cannot be seen except
through inward insight. Your reality is that inward
meaning. Everything else follows upon it.[1]

Inner insight is gained through self-examination. Self-
examination is defined as learning to balance accounts or
to be precise in calculating actions and thoughts in moving
towards their Lord because God also keeps account of
their action. The Quran says, "*And surely whether you manifest what is within you or keep it hidden, God will call you to
account for it*" (2:284). And, "*Oh you who believe, be aware of
God and look well into yourselves to see what you have in stock
for tomorrow*" (59:18).

Algazel, a well-known theologian and Sufi explains,

Just before going to sleep each night, the devotee
should take account of what his self (*nafs*) has done during the day so that his profits and losses get separated
from his investments. The investments here are the necessary actions (*wājib*); the profits are the recommended

(*mustahab*) actions; and the losses are those actions which have been prohibited (*ḥarām*). Just as one would purchase with care from a wily merchant, so must one bargain with caution in dealing with the self—for the self is a tricky and deceitful impostor that has a way of presenting its purposes in the garb of spiritual obedience so that one considers as profit what was really loss. In fact, in every action which is questionable, the devotee should examine his motivation carefully. If it is determined that the motivation came from the self, then compensation should be demanded of it.[2]

In order to come to know the self to know the Lord, one has to enter a world of correspondences. This refers not to the outer, quantitative form but the inner qualitative meaning of self. Meaning comes through being inner connected with the unity of nature. This inner connectedness produces a correspondence between the human being and the cosmos, both reflecting their Divine Origin. Correspondences are referred to as symbols or Signs as the Quran says:

> Have you not seen how God cites a symbol? A good word is as a good tree—its roots set firm and its branches in heaven, giving its fruit at every season by the leave of its Lord. So God cites symbols of human beings that they may remember (14:29-31).

To understand self, then, in the perspective of spiritual chivalry, it is necessary to understand the way the human being is viewed not only as the microcosmic mirror of the macrocosmic universe but how each of his or her component parts are but another correspondence relating back to the Divine Origin.

If the development of consciousness of self is not directed at this stage towards gaining knowledge of the Absolute and freely accepting the guidance of revelation, the self moves towards what is known as *kufr* to the spiritual warrior or ingratitude. This ingratitude may take the form of disbelief in the Oneness of God. It may also mean belief in a multiple of gods which is called *shirk* or multitheism or in pretending to believe in the Oneness of God by expressing it with one's tongue while one's heart sings a different tune and this is called *nifāq* or hypocrisy.

The goal of spiritual warriors is to return to their nature originated by God (belief in the oneness of God). With this as the goal, spiritual warriors become conscious of blessings, illumination and inner insights, freely choosing the guidance of revelation, therefore abandoning major wrongdoings and effecting self-reformation through good deeds towards others. They then become the pivot point for the manifestation of the ethics in society as its instrument. It is then that the return to their nature originated by God is in complete submission to the Will of God (*islām*) through actually experiencing it and not just observing it.

Those who are not aware of or who freely choose to reject Reality are considered by spiritual chivalry to be in moral imbalance. Here, the self, falls into a state of ignorance (*jahl*) of Reality because of having gone astray from their nature originated by God (*fiṭrat Allāh*). Those who are aware and freely choose to accept Reality are then able to move towards moral healing and the state of the moral reasonableness of a religiously cultured monotheist (*ḥilm*).

PART III
CAUSES OF
MORAL IMBALANCE

CHAPTER 1
INTRODUCTION

Moral imbalance results from the interaction of the processes of nature-nurture. Nature, as we have seen, provides the self with the ability to think and to feel and to act. When feeling and action are not ruled by reason (thinking), they develop negative traits and are called the passions. A nurturing environment may reinforce either. When it reinforces negative feelings and actions, it results in moral imbalance.

The causes of imbalance are clearly spelled out in the Quran and Traditions (*ahadiih*) for the spiritual warrior whose goal is to return to the nature originated by God. This nature is that of the unveiled spiritual heart, the inner Light within. This Light becomes veiled through a nurturing process that leads to moral imbalance and is unveiled through moral healing that results in moral balance.

While nature has provided a positive aspect of self— the moral reasonableness of a religiously cultured monotheist— at the level of thinking, to correct any imbalances gained through the nurturing process, it has also provided a negative aspect of self at the cognitive or thinking level which the spiritual warrior considers to be the main cause of imbalance: ignorance of Reality, the Truth. Moral reasonableness at the psychological level operates out of the ability to think positively of Reality while ignorance of Reality operates out of negative thinking, feelings or actions.

Descriptions of moral imbalance as provided by Shah Walīullāh help to further understand what the spiritual warrior sees. The way towards moral balance is to purify thoughts, feelings and actions through the spiritual method which God revealed without distinction to all of humanity, that is, regardless of gender, race or culture. This is the unity underlying all of human creation which is regulated by following both the Law and the Way as revealed to the Prophets.

At another level, reason is described as the spirit and its natural function is to preserve the possibility of eternal self. Feelings and actions together make up what is known as the passions. In psychological terms, they consist of the interaction of attraction to pleasure and avoidance of harm/pain. Attraction to pleasure is the basic instinct to preserve the species while avoidance of harm is the instinctive nature to preserve the individual.

Shah Walīullāh says,

> There is a type of person whose attraction to plea-sure, including that of sexual energy, is very strong but as far as his avoidance of pain and his thinking or rea-soning ability are concerned, the person is dull-minded. Anger, courage, fear and shame are slow to appear in him and they disappear in no time. His recollection of the past is as weak as is his capacity to plan for the future and decide what is positive and what is negative. Such a person is like a vegetable.
>
> A second kind of person shows courage and zeal, generosity and authority. In these qualities of actions, the person surpasses his companions but in his attrac-tion to pleasure function and reasoning powers, he hardly possesses a tenth of what others possess. He is like a wild beast.
>
> Yet a third type of person is one who distinguishes himself from those around him by his reasoning abili-ties, his capacity to restrain the attraction to pleasure function (based on positive feelings) but his avoidance of pain function does not follow. This is his weak spot. Such a person is comparable to the lower angels.
>
> In the case of the first person, reason or positive thinking is subservient to the attraction to pleasure func-

tion. The attraction to pleasure function is overdeveloped and therefore unreceptive to reason. This includes someone who indulges in inappropriate sexual pleasures outside the bounds of the Law or who is overly attentive to indulgence in gourmet food and drink. Even though the fear of the punishment for this may occur to him and his reason may vividly portray the abuse, humiliation and hatred which await him, he is just like a male ass falling upon a female or one that is bent on fodder. He takes no account at all of the negative effects, so engrossed is he in what he is doing. All of this makes people of common sense realize that every part is busy dominating as well as supporting the other. Reason may occasionally understand the baseness of the action and its negative consequences, but it cannot put its orders into effect.

It may also happen that the actions are filled with the desire for a lover and yet the necessary sexual energy is lacking in which case there is an underdevelopment of the attraction to pleasure function. Or the avoidance of pain function may be filled with contempt and vengeful thoughts and yet the arm lacks strength. Occasionally in such cases feelings arising from the attraction to pleasure come to the aid of the actions arising from the avoidance of harm/pain and pour in renewed vigor. This negative trait is also difficult to eradicate.

If, as with the second type, avoidance of harm is overdeveloped in trying to preserve the individual, and unreceptive to reason, acts of aggression become apparent. Besides a violent temper, the person tries to stay in control of situations, is ambitious and power hungry. This is an indication of the underdevelopment of the avoidance of harm/pain function. Sometimes reason may absorb knowledge calculated to further the drive for conquest. To this end it then begins to think out beneficial contingencies and effective plans, thus retreating from its former convictions. This is a negative trait which is extremely difficult to eradicate.

This person is such that when he becomes angry or jealous or is overtaken by worry or shame, his 'self' ceases to function. He feels neither hunger nor thirst and lacks even the strength to digest and evacuate. No matter how much his reason may chide him and tell him there is no point in showing anger or worrying, it is impossible for him to escape the dictates of his actions. Such a person has an underdeveloped avoidance of pain function.

When reason or thinking positively predominates, as with the third type, positive feelings or desires and actions result. As an example, when a person comes to realize through his reason that his happiness lies in keeping his instinct to preserve the species (attraction to pleasure) and to preserve the individual (avoidance of harm/pain) in moderation, then he no longer goes against or objects to the commands of reason. It often happens that a person of strong powers of reason thinks of some desirable worldly or religious objective. At that point, no matter how much his avoidance of harm may dislike certain aspects of it, and even though his attraction to pleasure function finds pleasures slipping through his hands, still his 'self' obeys reason.

These characteristics are like natural, physical needs. It is impossible to totally eradicate them. They may be temporarily concealed while severe spiritual exercises are being performed but no sooner are these spiritual exercises discontinued than they reappear once more. In fact the moral healing of these characteristics can only consist in this: that one uses them in their proper place, contenting oneself with what is necessary and avoiding excess. That is, that one learn to exercise justice towards the self.

To recapitulate briefly: the attraction to pleasure is located in the liver, the avoidance of harm is located in the physical heart, and reason is located in the brain. The attraction to pleasure permeates the whole body but is firmly rooted in the liver. The motivation to avoid harm is present throughout the whole body but it is firmly rooted in the heart and reason or thinking also pervades the entire body but it is firmly rooted in the brain. It should be borne in mind that God has created two distinct types of energy in the human being. One comprises the earthly, human energies, collectively called animal energy (the passions) by means of which the human being performs the actions of animals and is thus counted as one of them. The other type of energy comprises the spiritual faculties by means of which the human being carries out the work of angels and is hence regarded as one of their number.[1]

The meaning and purpose of the moral healing of the self is that the spiritual energy should gain control over the animal energy and that the characteristics of the former should come into prominence while those of the animal should remain in abeyance with a corresponding decrease in their effects. Shah Walīullāh adds, however, that this is not easy to understand.

Since there are so many variations in the three basic types of human being, the means of moral healing for each of them will also differ. Thus the scope of this topic becomes enormous. It should be remembered, too, that the stages of moral healing of these three types are also different. Each has its own form and pattern. This is why the matter has become obscure and bewildering to a number of spiritual warriors who are unable to understand how to effect unity among all the multiplicity of forms and patterns of the three types. However, there are people who do recognize and distinguish all the different forms and patterns and are well-acquainted with the method of achieving a systematic and consistent unity for 'God speaks the Truth and shows the Way'.[2]

CHAPTER 2
PASSIONS VS. REASON

In terms of psychology, the greater struggle is described by the Sufis between reason and the passions for the attention of the heart.

REASON

Al-Muḥāsibī defines reason as a natural disposition or instinct bestowed by God upon His creatures. It is invisible to them both within themselves and/or in others. It can be neither tasted nor touched nor experienced yet it is the means through which God made them to know Him. It is through reason that they bear witness to Him. It is through reason that they recognize what is positive and beneficial and what is negative and harmful. Anyone who can distinguish between these two has proof that God gave him reason. Al-Muḥāsibī says, "The Sign of it is the power to organize and to put things in their right place, whether in speech or in act, and the proof of that is the preference of the greater good to the lesser."[1]

According to spiritual chivalry, reason is a natural instinct which uses experience to obtain knowledge. It is a blessing from God to be able to understand the revelation and through its guidance, learning to read its Signs, one becomes a believer. This view is based on a Divine Tradition which says,

By My Majesty and My Glory and My Greatness and My Power and My Sovereignty over My Creation, I have not created any being for which I have greater regard or which is more precious to Me than you or more excellent in My Sight than you are in your dignity because through you I am known and through you I am

> worshiped and by means of you I am praised and
> through you I take and by you I give and by you I
> requite. To you I give My reward and upon you comes
> My chastisement.[2]

It is through reason as defined by Ibn al-'Arabī as a
state in constant fluctuation that the believer comes to
understand the Unity of God, not in the sense of actually
experiencing it but in the sense of reflecting upon It.
Through reflection based on reason, the human being has
been empowered by God to understand His counseling to
the positive (commands) and prevention of the negative
(prohibitions) by healing the self. God's commands and
prohibitions spell out the duties and obligations of the
trustee. These include counseling the self to that which
God has commanded and preventing the self from that
which God has prohibited (*amr bi'l ma'rūf wa nahy an al-
munkar*). A person who manifests moral reasonableness is
obedient to his or her Lord for any disobedience shows a
lack of ability to reason because reason is the means
through which God speaks to the conscience of His servants. He speaks through promises and warnings so that
they can learn to discriminate between what is morally
positive and negative, what is both harmful and beneficial
in this world and the next.

Again, a Tradition confirms this for the spiritual warrior:

> God will not accept the prayers of a person or his
> fasting or his pilgrimage or his giving of alms or his
> warfare for the sake of God (*jihād*) or anything in the
> nature of good works, if he has not used in reason (to
> understand the true significance of these things).[3]

It is reason which is convinced by having facts presented to it. Al-Muḥāsībī points out that if reason is rightly

directed, it is one of the greatest blessings of God.[4]

There is no adornment like that of reason and no garment wherewith a person is clothed more fair than knowledge for God Most High is not known except by means of reason and is not obeyed except through knowledge. Every good and perfect gift he holds comes from God but it is for the human being to make the best possible use of such gifts and he is to employ his reason in order to co-operate with the grace of God. Know that the origin of every speech is action (that is, of the heart) and the origin of every action is knowledge and the origin of all that is, is the grace of God (*tawfiq*) combined with the right use of the intelligence and much reflection.[5]

If the nurturing process does not reinforce the strengthening of one's ability to reason, reason will fail to be guided by revelation, fail to prefer moral reasonableness to wrongdoing, fail to choose knowledge rather than to remain in ignorance of Reality.

THE PASSIONS

When the natural ability to reason is not reinforced by the nurturing process, the self automatically falls into the other natural force within and that is what is known as "the passions." As has been pointed out, the passions are known as the animal aspects of self. While animal qualities are good for animals and for basic instinctive drives like the preservation of the species or the individual, they have a negative effect if they rule the human being. When they rule, the human being no longer listens to the counsel of reason.

The tension between the natural ability to reason in order to preserve the eternal possibility of self and the natural animal qualities of attraction to pleasure and avoidance of harm is present as long as life is present. The greater struggle for the spiritual warrior, as we have seen, is to turn the self away from the animal within towards the spirit within, the higher aspect of human nature. This battle takes place within what is known as the heart.

While reason urges the heart to turn inward, towards the connectedness of self with the Source, with that which unites all of nature, the passions, as the lower aspect of human nature, urges the heart to turn towards the outer senses and physical members of the body. Consisting as the passions do of attraction to pleasure and avoidance of harm, the desires of the physical members as fed by the outer senses conflict with God's Law. They strive after their own interests regardless of what is pleasing to God or due to their fellow human beings. It is a state which is unreceptive to Divine Grace, being wilful and headstrong in obeying the animal qualities of self. Al-Muḥāsībī says,

> Place the animal self (*nafs ammārah*, the passions) where God Almighty placed it. Describe it as He has described it. Withstand it according to His command for it is a greater enemy to you than Satan himself. Satan gains power over you only by means of it and your consent to it. You know to what it calls you and that it was created weak, though its nature is strong in greed and deceit, for it is self-confident, self-assertive, disobedient to God, untrustworthy. Its sincerity consists in lying. Its claims are based on vanity. All that comes from it is deceitful. Nothing that it does is praiseworthy. Be not deluded by the self and its hopes and its desires for if you leave it alone, you are led astray and if you give it what it desires, you will perish. If you neglect to examine it, you will fall under its control. If you weaken in your struggles against it, you will be overwhelmed. If you follow it in its desires, you will go down into hell. The truth is not in it nor any tendency to good. It is the source of affliction, the origin of all evil and the trea-

sure-house of Iblis. None knows it save its Creator—
what it displays as fear is really self-confidence and
what it displays as sincerity is only falsehood. Its claim
to be single-minded in the service of God is pure
hypocrisy.[6]

The animal self (*nafs ammārah*), the passions, then,
direct the heart towards wrongdoing, away from the
duties and responsibilities of the self as a trustee of nature,
turning the self, instead, into the rebellious self, the idol
within.

Like an animal which is at first wild and untamed,
the animal self must be trained by constant discipline in
order to become of use to him who is its master so that
he, in his turn, may carry out the Will of the greater
Master, his Lord. Since this discipline will mean the ulti-
mate salvation of the self as part of the whole person, it
is an act of compassion towards it. Slowly and reluctant-
ly the self may be brought under obedience. From time
to time it will still struggle against the compulsion
brought to bear upon it. It will continue to seek. It will
try to get out from being disciplined. The constant pres-
sure brought to bear against it by degrees will subdue it.
This, in turn, will allow the spiritual aspect of the heart,
the reproachful self (*nafs lawwāmah*), to gain the upper-
hand. When the reproachful self (reason, thinking, cognition) gains control of the animal self (*nafs ammārah*)
wins the struggle, the battle is over and victory of the
spiritual heart is achieved. Iblis and his hosts have been
routed and the lusts of the flesh no longer make any
appeal; the animal self has become a captive, in complete submission to the Will of its Lord. It has become
the soul at rest (*nafs al-muṭma'innah*).[7]

When the passions rule, there is a weakening of the
cognitive function or the ability to reason. The spiritual

heart is veiled and cognition or reason makes decisions based on ignorance of the Reality. The person is viewed by the spiritual warrior as being led by their own lusts, unjust and morally imbalanced, not rightly guided, heedless and disobedient to the Commander-in-Chief, unworthy of the trust, in rebellion against the covenant.

There are three situations possible in this struggle of reason vs. the passions based on the verse, *"But there are among them (Our servants) some who wrong their own self; some who are just; and some who are the foremost of those who are near to God"* (35:32). *"Those who wrong themselves,"* according to spiritual chivalry are those in whom the the passions dominate. The second, *"those who are just,"* are those in whom reason dominates leading to *murūwwah* or *futuwwah* and the third, *"the foremost of those who are near to God,"* are those who have passed through the middle course (morally healed) where reason rules over the passions and then, aided by Divine Grace, move towards the domination of self through intuition. This leads to *walāyah* or sanctity, being a friend of God.

If the passions rule, the passions or animal aspect of self prevails and so subdues the power of reason that reasonableness rarely surfaces. The person so dominated by the passions is untrustworthy. If the passions continue to grow stronger and reason weaker, the person becomes a hypocrite which will be described further on.

If reason rules, reason holds the passions in check but they are still very much alive. As long as reasonableness is strong in the person, the person is among those who are just and are called *"Companions of the Right"* (90:18).

> *And what will explain to you the path that is steep? It is the freeing of a slave, or giving food upon a day of hunger to an orphan or a near of kin or a needy person in misery; then that he becomes of those who believe and counsel each other to be patient and counsel each other to be merciful. Those are the Companions of the Right Hand* (90:11-18).

If the furthest development of reason or intuition rules, then the person is able to permanently starve the passions. These people are known as *"the foremost of those who are near to God"* (35: 32).

CHAPTER 3
IGNORANCE (*jahl*) OF REALITY

For the spiritual warrior, people who ignore their nature originated by God, their natural belief in the oneness of God (*tawḥid*), who are ruled by their passions, are in a state of ignorance of Reality. In the view of spiritual chivalry, they are people who, although originally created with this inner or innate knowledge, have allowed the nurturing process to cover over this truth, manifesting negligence, heedlessness and/or forgetfulness. Rather than expressing themselves towards others through a state of the moral reasonableness of a religiously cultured monotheist (*ḥilm*), they relate to themselves and to others through this state of ignorance (*jahl*) of Reality. Instead of relating to the world in a state of harmony, balance and equilibrium, they foster oppression, discrimination, prejudice, intolerance and injustice.

This ignorance manifests itself in certain cognitive, affective and behavioral patterns which are clearly evident of them having forgotten their original nature, their heart, their covenant with their Lord, their being potentially the trustee of nature and God's vicegerent on earth.

Behavioral patterns arising out of a state of ignorance of Reality may appear occasionally or be so entrenched that they become habitual. One of the major manifestations that the spiritual warrior guards against is that of tribal or family honor. This trait manifests itself in zeal for what the person thinks must be defended at all costs. The person jealously guards his tribal or family honor and take pride in it. If the person's honor is tarnished, compromised or violated, the person responds with moral indignation, stern protest and angry resistance.

Manifesting a resistance to criticism, even if it be fair,

the person builds up a shield against submitting to anyone or anything including Reality. Anything that humiliates or humbles the person in the slightest way is responded to with scorn and disdain. Without regard to positive or negative, right or wrong, anyone who is under the person's protection is defended and everyone else is considered to be inferior.

The pride in themselves and their family that develops out of this state of ignorance is referred to as rebellion (against God's Commands) and arrogance in the Quran.[1] They feel themselves to be Lord of themselves, liberated and a servant of no one—human or Divine. To the spiritual warrior, what a person in this state fails to recognize is that by refusing to consciously return to their original nature as servant (*'abd*) to the Lord (*rabb*) alone, they become the slave of their own ego. They are free to make this choice, but the freedom and liberation they sense is illusory. They are still worshipping something because the concept of worship is part of their innate or original nature and *"there is no changing of God's creation"* (30:30). They have, however, gone astray. Instead of worshipping the One, the Absolute, the Truth, the Reality, they worship their own ego which is relative to themselves alone. Therefore a presumptuousness, insolence and arrogance develops out of this pride in this human power. An arrogant self-confidence results instead of the natural state of submission to the One Creator.

> *While the disbelievers set an arrogant self-confidence in their hearts—the arrogance of ignorance—God sent down His tranquility upon His Messenger and the believers and made them stick closely to the command of self-restraint...(48:26).*

At the level of feelings and actions, the state of ignorance of Reality expresses itself in outbursts of passion.

With this loss of temper at the slightest provocation, they become uncontrollable. The consequences of this impetuous and hasty behavior is recklessness. Without any reflection, acting out of their uncontrolled emotional state, violent behavior often ensures. They lose a sense of what is right and wrong. It flows up in their heart, disturbs their balance of mind, makes them lose sight of positive and negative reactions and drives them to destructive actions.

Ignorance of Reality at the thinking level also has severe consequences for one's natural sense of morality according to spiritual chivalry. The state of ignorance weakens the natural power of the human mind to reason leading to injustice. This results in shallow rash judgments. One loses the capacity to take exact measure of self, to know the natural limitations of one's ability. As a result, one tends to go beyond the natural bounds. In this state, the mind's ability to understand God's Will behind the veil of the manifest world is incapacitated. One loses sight of natural events as God's Signs and even the most self-evident of truths become veiled, covered over.

INJUSTICE
GOING BEYOND GOD'S BOUNDS

The Quran establishes the duties and obligations of human conduct in society which the spiritual warrior sees as being the conditions for becoming the trustee. They are called "God's bounds" (*hūdūd Allāh*). Those who remain within God's bounds will be rewarded and those who go beyond the bounds will be punished. Those who transgress the bounds are known as "oppressors" (*ẓalimun*). *"All those who transgress the bounds of God, they are the oppressors"* (2:229). A person may also oppress themselves. *"....whoso transgresses God's bounds has oppressed himself"* (65:1).

To go beyond God's bounds is any kind of human act

that goes beyond the proper limit and encroaches on the rights of others. It is to hurt someone seriously without any just cause. The spiritual warrior hears the warning:

> Drive not away those who call upon their Lord at morning and evening desiring His Presence (Face). No responsibility for them is upon you and no responsibility for you is upon them that you should drive them away and become one of the oppressors (6:52).

To go to excess is to be unjust. "*Oh believers, do not make unlawful the good things which God has made lawful for you, but commit no excess. Verily God loves not those given to excess*" (5:87). Going beyond God's bounds, an aspect of the negative state of injustice, is seen in spiritual chivalry as being rebellious. It also means to exceed or transgress the right measure. It carries an unmistakable implication of enmity, aggressiveness or encroachment upon another's rights. It is to behave too extravagantly and to be immoderate, to commit excesses. "*He it is Who produces gardens trellised as well as untrellised, the date-palm and crops of various tastes and olives and pomegranates alike and unlike. Eat you of the fruit thereof when they fructify and bring the due thereof upon the harvest day but commit not extravagance. Verily He loves not the extravagant*" (6:14).

To be an oppressor basically means to put things in the wrong place. It means to act in such a way as to transgress the proper limit and encroach upon the right of some other person. It is to do injustice in the sense of going beyond the bounds and doing what one has no right to do because God declares that He Himself does not do this. "*I do absolutely no wrong to My servants*" (50:29). While God does not wrong anyone '*even by the weight of an ant*' (4:49) or '*by a single date-thread*' (4:40) the human being does.

Oppression may be from the human being to God or from human being to human being. In the first, it consists of the human being's transgressing the limits of human conduct imposed by God Himself while in the second, it is to go beyond the bounds of proper conduct in social life recognized as such by society.

FOLLOWING PASSIONS

Following one's own passions and desires is to manifest conjectures concerning God and His revelation.[2] It turns moral-seekers away from the objective truth.[3] The person can end up taking his or her own ego as a god:

> *Have you not seen him who has taken his passions for his god and God has led him astray knowingly and has set a seal upon his hearing and his heart and has placed a covering upon his eyesight? Who shall then guide him after God? (45:23). There succeeded them (the great Prophets such as Abraham, Moses, Ishmael, etc.) a generation who abandoned the prayer and followed their passions (19:59). And who is more astray than one who follows his own passions devoid of guidance from God (28:50).*

DISBELIEF (kufr)

Kufr means to cover in the sense of to knowingly ignore the benefits one has received and therefore to be ungrateful. This denial of Reality manifests itself in various acts of insolence, haughtiness and presumptuousness. Therefore, *kufr* is the exact opposite of humbleness and clashes with the idea of fear of God.

Disbelief may arise from not learning to read God's Signs.

> *Oh people of the Book! Why do you disbelieve in the Signs of God when you yourself bear witness to them? (3:70). Have not the disbelievers then beheld that the heavens and the earth were a mass all sewn up and then We unstiched them and of water fashioned every living thing? Will they not*

believe? And We set in the earth firm mountains lest it should shake with them, and We set in it ravines to serve as ways, that haply so they may be guided; and We set up the heaven as a roof well-protected; yet still from Our Signs they are turning away. It is He who created the night and the day, the sun and the moon, each swimming in a sky (21:30-33).

Veiled by ignorance of Reality, they cannot accept the Signs and believe in the One God.

INGRATITUDE

God sometimes gives a very detailed list of the Signs (blessings) which He has bestowed upon people[4] and adds that in spite of such blessings on His part, most people remain negligent of the duty to be grateful to Him. God does not expect the human being to be grateful for all the blessings but the majority of people are ungrateful.[5]

VEILED HEARTS

The heart of the disbeliever is veiled[6] or sealed[7] or has rust covering it.[8] Those who have a heart[9] should easily grasp the deep meaning of God's Signs. The revealed words of God should work as a reminder. But being veiled and obstructed, the hearts of the disbelievers cannot perceive the religious significance of anything.

Having a veiled heart, the disbeliever cannot apprehend the Signs of God as they are even though he gives ear to the recitation of the Quran and looks towards the Prophet. To him, the Divine Signs are just fairy tales of old folks.[10]

HYPOCRISY (*nifāq*)

The principle of all talk, no action, lip service followed by betrayal through behavior are characteristic of the hypocrite. They are faithless to any bond or treaty they have made.[11]

There are three basic types of hypocrite according to Shah Walīullāh.

First there is the type of person who is ruled by his passions. Both his actions and his reason are subservient to his feelings. His aggressive actions and perceptive reasoning ability lend them their support. By nature such a person goes wherever he likes without the permission of law or reason and does whatever he wishes. He becomes involved in love affairs even though reason and the Law forbid it. If he is held up to shame by conventional standards, he pays this no heed whatsoever as if he had some kind of certificate exempting him from the Law and from popular retribution. He always keeps in mind some excuse or other for his behavior and uses this to drive out any thought for the Law which may be lurking like a last grain of faith in the back of his mind. In the Quran God describes such a hypocrite as deceitful. '*They try to deceive God but He deceives them.*' (4:142). Elsewhere there is reference to their 'twisted breasts' (11:5). By breast is meant the knowledge of the breast. The twisting of it means that the hypocrite covers the thought of truth with the thought of untruth and changes his knowledge into ignorance.

Sometimes this type of hypocrite sinks even lower than this and does not take the slightest note of the Law, being entirely satisfied with his unspoken excuse although at times conflict and contradiction may flare up in his breast. Or he may sink still lower and, holding firmly to his sense of license, become totally indifferent to the prohibition of the Law. Occasionally he may sink to the lowest level of all and actually begin to take pride in his wrongdoing and try to demonstrate its beauty. In such a case as God has said, '*Their wrongdoing has encompassed them. They are the companions of the fire and will remain there forever.*' (2:81).

This type of person plunges himself into such indulgences (attracted as he is to pleasure) including over-eat-
ing (gluttony) and setting animals to fight one another.
He enjoys ease and fine living and forever craves splendid clothes and finely decorated houses. The very
thought of these things gives him pleasure. His heart
takes delight in seeking them. Even his intellect is likewise engaged in striving for them. He is angry with
those who criticize such activities and takes as his friend
whoever approves of his pursuits. He shows aversion
towards everything which tends to keep him away from
his pleasures. Where friendship is concerned, he spends
his wealth lavishly and gives freely of himself to help
any friend in need. Conversely, if he has occasion to
show hatred, he thinks nothing of abusing, striking or
even killing the offending person. He may keep a
grudge concealed for a long time but in the end it will
come into the open. His intellect uses every possible
device to conjure up the image of pleasure and it thinks
up stratagems to obtain it. It removes any obstacles from
his path and grants him license in anything he might
consider himself unable to do.

The second type of hypocrite is one whose aggressive energy (avoidance of harm/pain) is excessive with
the result that his 'self' and his intellect are subservient.
Such a person is constantly engaged in gaining domi-
nance over his fellows and revenging himself on those
who put up any resistance. He can conceal a grudge for
a long time and is continuously thinking of killing, striking, overthrowing or humiliating his adversaries. He
accepts those who defer to him and seeks to overthrow
anyone who happens to be his equal. The slightest word
is enough to make him lose his temper and declare that
he is not the sort of person who can brook any dishonor
or threat. 'Come what may, its all the same to me. Rather
hell-fire than dishonor!' Such is his religion. It is also
part of his religion to go to extremes in the pursuit of his
honor. In this respect his self obeys him and his intellect

assists him. He is prepared to tolerate any hardship if he can thereby give practical expression to his anger. With the greatest ease he devises plans to show his rancor and revenge.

Sometimes, on the other hand, he may be seized with such a degree of friendship for people or attachment to a custom that he strives valiantly on their behalf without considering the prohibitions of the Law and reason. It is an essential feature of his conduct, so he says, to remain loyal to his friends and it is an inherent part of his constitution to abide by his own customs. He is not one of those shameless creatures who can change friends and customs from one moment to the next. In the opinion of the uninformed, such people with a marked aggressive drive, are truly strong and superior to those who are driven by feelings, in particular, their extreme form of lust. However, tastes differ.

The third type of hypocrite is one whose intelligence is confused. Or perhaps his intellect may be sound but he has nonetheless fallen into some sort of error—such as believing that God has a body or ascribing human attributes to God or believing that God does not have any attributes, etc. Or he may entertain doubts concerning the Quran or the Prophet or the future life without ever having gone so far as to be declared an apostate.

Alternatively the situation may be that his intelligence has been overrun by dark oppressive thoughts so that he is no longer convinced about anything and is thus unable to bring his intentions to any sort of conclusion. Or it may be that he has gone too deeply into poetry or mathematics and thus failed to give sufficiently deep thought to the Law.[12]

MULTITHEISM (*shirk*)

Multitheism is another type of disbelief to the spiritual warrior who also considers it to be caused by ignorance of Reality. It lies in the belief that other forces besides God have a role to play in directing the affairs of the world. If one worships these forces, the spiritual warrior calls it multitheism in worship and if one obeys these forces, it is called multitheism in obedience. Multitheism in worship is also referred to as manifest multitheism by the spiritual warrior while multitheism in obedience is referred to as hidden multitheism.

A multitheist of either type is compared in the Quran to a person who stretches forth his hands in vain towards the mirage of water in the desert[13] or as a person covered by thick layers of darkness on a vast, abysmal sea.[14]

It manifests itself in oppression,[15] extravagance,[16] haughtiness or arrogance.[17] It is to deny the Signs much like a disbeliever.[18]

It can also manifest itself in violence and outrage,[19] pride,[20] contentiousness,[21] envy,[22] and inappropriate anger.[23]

PART IV
OBSERVING MORAL BALANCE
IN NATURE

CHAPTER 1
LEARNING TO READ THE SIGNS

The spiritual warrior obtains moral balance, the stage of *murūwwah*, through rigorous self-examination. Self-examination is enhanced by the spiritual warrior through the Sign of the Presence of God, as proof of God's Presence in the microcosm and the macrocosm.

Self-examination begins by learning to read the Signs. He or she understands the verse, *"We shall show them Our Signs upon the horizon and within themselves until it is clear to them that it is the Real (the Truth),"* (41:53) as expressing the view that Signs of the Presence of God are expressed in both the macrocosmic universe and the microcosmic human being. Each of them—the outer forms and the inner meaning—are themselves works of "sacred art," not only as forms but as meaningful forms. The purpose for each of them reflects the eternal beauty that lives within all of creation. It is this eternal beauty, the inner meaning, which connects the microcosmic human being, the only being in which God directly blew His Spirit, the only being created in His image, to the unity and oneness of all of nature.

The self as microcosm, reflecting all that is contained in the macrocosm in terms of meaning can be transformed into the same moral goodness everything else in nature contains. It has been provided with the ability to perfect itself by nature's processes (God's Will). While nature itself perfects everything except the human being through the natural processes, the human being, having free-will, can choose to do as nature does.

IMITATING NATURE'S PROCESSES

For the moral healer who historically has been a member of the craft guilds committed to creating the music, art and architecture of the traditional world, as well as a member of a traditional athletic association, member of a neighborhood watch group, or as knight to the One King (Malik al-Mulk), this choice is to imitate the creative process as it naturally unfolds in nature. This imitation, however, is not in a competitive sense or in an arrogant sense to try to outdo nature, but in a humble sense, in a sense of complete submission to God's Will.

Spiritual warriors observe nature. They see that nature is completely submissive to God's Will, to the natural processes. They then realize that something is holding them back from being able to submit as nature does. That which is holding them back is the idol/ego within created through a nurturing process that develops ignorance of the Real instead of moral reasonableness because of the Real; that shows ingratitude (*kufr*) to the Real for life and a chance to consciously choose to perfect self instead of thankfulness for this blessing; that develops a disbelief (*kufr*) in the One Who created them instead of belief in that One God; that develops a belief in more than One God (*shirk*) not recognizing that if it were Real, the universe would be based in chaos and not order, harmony, equilibrium and balance; that develops a seeming belief in the One God with words while the heart holds a different belief (*nifāq*).

The moral response of spiritual warriors is that of the trustees of nature and self, of the macrocosm and the microcosm. As trustees, they allow self, freely and consciously, to choose to become an instrument for the trust. Recognizing that they do not have the power to create the trust, they give that power to something whose will is All-Will and whose power is All-Power instead of trying to take over the position of Trust-Giver.

NATURE'S TRUSTEE

Imitating the processes of nature, then, spiritual warriors first submit to the processes in order to gain the qualifications to become a trustee. The qualifications are laid out in the ethics of the Law and the Way.

The word used in this context is that of *ḥanīf* which essentially means to be a monotheist. In order to become a monotheist, conscious of the trust, they must learn to control all impulses that could be considered idolatry by the Trust-Maker. The greatest idol to overcome is that of ego— the self that develops through the nurturing process. This idol is controlled by reason. To be in control of the idol within is to have gained the moral reasonableness of a person cultured by monotheism (*ḥilm*). At this point one can be called a spiritual warrior who has passed through the stage of moral goodness (*murūwwah*).

It is then that the Work as a re-creator of "sacred art"— self/ artist/ artisan/ architect/athlete/lower angel begins. The "Work" is to return the material at hand—the natural self, is striving towards moral healing, yarn if carpet weaving, stucco if builder, silver if silversmith, gold if goldsmith and so forth—to its spiritual origin. By imitating the processes of nature within the context of being a trustee, a vicegerent, the worker uses his or her breath through chanting, invocation, or rhythmic breathing or counting to unveil the material's inner meaning. This inner meaning accompanies the outer form created so that it becomes "something more than the sum of its parts."

Just as the universe is conceived of as having been created through the Divine Breath, so the artist / artisan / architect / athlete / lower angel enlivens the natural forms at his or her disposal with the eternal beauty which resides within each form. The breath, whether it be the Divine Breath which creates the universe and sustains it, or the breath of the monotheist (*ḥanīf*), morally reasonable (*ḥalīm*) spiritual warrior *(fatā/fatāt)* is what is known as Divine Grace (*barakah*).

The Presence of the One God in the universe presupposes an order, balance and harmony in nature. Nature in its mode of operation unfolds in a unified and harmonic way. The unity of nature is that it is able to unite the inner and the outer, the hidden and the manifest. The language is that of pattern, pattern based on numbers and geometry. In the traditional view, the patterns of the macrocosm are moved by the same Divine Source that moves the microcosmic self. By the self being in harmony with them, by centering the self on the same hidden Vertical Axis that they are centered, on a sense of oneness and unity develops between them.

Traditional humanity views all of creation as emanation from the One. This interconnectedness means that human beings share with nature a commonalty of structure that is expressed through mathematical laws of similitude, symmetry and geometry.

> The harmonic order and sense of unity observed in a snow crystal depends as much on its geometrical order as on its ability to reflect a higher and more profound order. All shapes, surfaces and lines in nature are arranged in conformity to a geometric order inherent in nature and reflect the ideal systems of oneness. Resting on the objective foundation, independent of the human being's subjective tastes, an order and harmony is attained that is general, universal and eternal. Order is viewed as a cosmic law whose processes the human being undertakes to comprehend through arithmetic, geometry and harmony. Proportion is to space what rhythms is to line and harmony to sound.[1]

Symbols or Signs of God upon the horizon and within themselves awaken the spiritual warrior to the Signs. The proof of transformation comes in the re-creations— whether they be the self or an object outside of self. If the human artist-creator has received the Grace, that Grace will be transferred to the object created. The object will then have earned the name "sacred art." It will reflect the Reality contained within the nature of things.

Symbols can be divided into universal or particular. Universal or natural symbols are as they appear in the nature of things. They represent, in a sense, the hidden or intrinsic sciences taught through oral tradition like the sciences of numbers, geometry, letters, spiritual alchemy and spiritual astrology. The study of universal symbols are also the subject of the extrinsic sciences like the traditional science of ethics. The former study both the "...the Signs upon the horizon...and within themselves" (41:53) while the latter relates to the self of the human form as "...the Signs within themselves..." (41:53). Particular symbols, on the other hand, vary from tradition to tradition. They may take either the form of a sensible object or an idea or concept which God consecrates through revelation to become instruments of Divine Grace (barakah).

NUMBERS

The spiritual warrior considers the sacred character of the first of God's revelations—the created order—to be the means through which God manifests multiplicity as so many reflections of Unity. The Quran says, "Nothing is there but its measures are with Us and We send it not down but in a known measure" (15:21). Beginning with numbers, they are important in the traditional perspective because through numbers the spiritual warrior is able to relate multiplicity to Unity and bring to light the harmony which pervades the Universe, developing what has been called "Abrahamic Pythagoreanism" because of the emphasis upon unity and oneness (Abrahamic) and the qualitative as well as the quantitative aspect of numbers (Pythagoreanism).

Comparing the relation of God to the world as that of One to other numbers, the Brethren of Purity (10th century) say in regard to the science of numbers that it is "the way leading to the grasp of Unity as a science which stands above Nature and is the principle of beings..."[2]

It is important to note,

> Numbers in Abrahamic Pythagoreanism being both qualitative and quantitative cannot be identified as modern numbers with simply division and multiplication because numbers are a projection of unity, never separated from their Source. They integrate the entity that they symbolize or with which they are identified with Unity, the Source of all existence.[3]

The Brethren of Purity say,

> All that has by nature and with systematic method been arranged in the Universe seems both in part and as a whole to have been determined and ordered in accordance with number by the forethought and mind of Him that created all things; for the pattern was fixed, like a preliminary sketch, by the domination of number pre-existing in the mind of the world-creating God, number conceptual only and immaterial in every way so that with reference to it, as to an artistic plan, should be created all these things, times, motion, the heavens, the stars and all sorts of revolution.[4]

Numbers as the fundamental ordering principles of nature have both a qualitative and quantitative significance. Their qualitative significance is their psychological aspect, the aspect involved in the processes of nature. Traditional numerology is synchronistic, non-linear and non-logical. Numbers are part of the Signs *"upon the hori-*

zons and within themselves." Reading numbers in this sense becomes equivalent to a kind of language.

A Sufi writes,

> Know that the wise Pythagoras was the first to discouse on the nature of number. He said beings come into existence in conformity with the nature of number. Consequently, he who understand the nature of number, its species and properties, is in a position to know the various genera and species of beings. Necessarily, things are one with respect to Matter and multiple with respect to Form. There must be dyads (matter and form, the subtle and the gross, the luminous and the dark, etc.); triads (surface, line and volume; past, future and present, etc.); tetrads (the four natures, the four elements, the four pillars of the cosmic tent); there must be pentads, hexads, heptads, decads, etc. ....Pythagoras and his followers...dispensed justice where justice was due. They saw very clearly that the One is the cause of number and that all numbers, small or big, even or odd, are constituted by the One. The One gives its name to every number; number persists because the One persists; number grows and augments by the repetition of the One. It is because a dyad is a dyadic unity, for example, that it is different from a triadic unity, and so on.[5]

GEOMETRY

Geometry expresses the personality of numbers permitting the human being a further exploration into the processes of nature.

> ...the triangle and the square are 'personalities' and not qualities. They are essentials and not accidents. While one obtains ordinary numbers by addition, qualitative number results, on the contrary, from an internal or intrinsic differentiation of principal unity; it is not added to anything and does not depart from unity.

Geometrical figures are so many images of unity; they exclude one another or rather, they denote different principal quantities; the triangle is harmony, the square stability; these are 'concentric' and not 'serial' numbers.'[6]

Al-Bīrūnī expresses the harmony of nature and the role of numbers and geometry in this harmony:

...Among the peculiarities of the flowers there is one really astonishing fact, viz., the number of their leaves, the tops of which form a circle when they begin to open, is in most cases conformable to the laws of geometry. In most cases they agree with the chords that have been found by the laws of geometry, not with conic sections. You scarcely ever find a flower of 7 or 9 leaves, for you cannot construct them according to the laws of geometry in a circle as isosceles [triangles]. The number of their leaves is always 3 or 4 or 5 or 6 or 18. This is a matter of frequent occurrence. Possibly one may find among the species hitherto known such a number of leaves, but, on the whole, one must say Nature preserves its genera and species such as they are. For if you would, for example, count the number of seeds of one of the many pomegranates of a tree, you would find that all the other pomegranates contain the same number of seeds as that one the seeds of which you have counted first. So, too, Nature proceeds in all other matters.[7]

THE SELF

A further universal symbol for the spiritual warrior is the human form itself which through the creative process can be transformed into the same moral goodness everything else in nature symbolizes. Spiritual warriors begin with self and then to their particular craft. Through the use of the breath—in the same way that the universe is conceived of having been created—they return a form to its origin. Spiritual warriors use the science of spiritual alchemy first in transforming self and then in transforming the matter and material of their craft. Spiritual astrology as the macrocosmic counterpart of spiritual alchemy, is referred to by spiritual warriors not as a means to predict future events but as a means to understand the Signs of God's Presence in the universe. This understanding, however, in the view of spiritual chivalry, can only come in a context free of the idol/ego.

For the Way, nature is an object of contemplation not simply to be observed but more importantly to be experienced. Experiencing nature means coming to know the inner workings of nature in a direct way and this can only be done by the human being coming to know self. The traditional method is to develop the moral reasonableness of a religiously cultured monotheist (ḥilm) and the model is that of spiritual chivalry.

The Quran divides all human qualities into positive and negative qualities. The final measure for the spiritual warrior is the belief in the One God, the Creator of all being. The Quran refers to the greater struggle between the development of positive traits as opposed to the negative. The struggle as mentioned there is between the monotheist, submissive to God's will, servant-believer who has unveiled the inner Light of the nature originated by God and the ungrateful disbeliever who may even believe in more than one god or pretend to believe with words while deeds show a different belief. While this struggle throughout history has occurred on the outside, for the spiritual warrior it begins within, in the inward dimension of self, through first moral healing the self. Once the warrior is morally healed, he or she has earned the title of trustee of nature given by the one Trust-Giver.

Morality is dealt with in the traditional science of ethics. The science of ethics, originating in the scientific method of observation of human nature developed parallel to the experiential lab-oratories of the orders of spiritual chivalry. While the importance of self-examination was still passed on through oral tradition as one of the key practices for moral healing, the geometric Sign of the Presence of God took the practice out of the oral tradition into the realm of self-help so that each potential spiritual hero or heroine could move through the practice of self-examination towards moral healing in a more independent fashion.

After striving through strenuous self-examination to heal morally, to develop moral goodness (*murūwwah*), sensing the need for further progress on the spiritual Way, some seek out a master while others feel content with at least trying to morally heal. Those who seek out a spiritual master, imperative to further spiritual development, are those who then have the potential for becoming future spiritual masters. Those who stop at the stage of moral healing, itself a tremendous inner battle, become active in social, political, economic, athletic and intellectual affairs in Islamic societies.

According to Gaston Bachelard, a contemporary thinker, proof of the soundness and validity of an idea or concept is when it can be conceptualized into a geometric form. The Sign the Sufis call "the Presence of God," better known in the West as the Enneagram, serves as proof of the soundness and validity of moral healing. It not only expresses the theoretical and practical microcosmic level of the inner self but has a macrocosmic counterpart as well, to be discussed next.

It is within the context of traditional Islam where emphasis is upon both the Law and the Way that understanding has to begin. From that context and its vital components of spiritual hermeneutics (*ta'wil*) of the language of symbolism, comes further realizations of the important individual and social implications of spiritual chivalry.

Following this comes respect for the traditional science of correspondences between the microcosmic human self and the macrocosmic universe.

Known as the science of balance, the science of spiritual alchemy is one of the key sciences underlying spiritual chivalry but it does not act alone. It is one partner in a mystical marriage with the science of psychoethics. Speaking the same symbolic language of the sciences of numbers and geometry, their earthly union mirrors a heavenly correspondence, that of spiritual astrology. The concept behind the Sign of "the Presence of God" is both in the heavens and within ourselves as so many signs confirming yet again the verse, *"We shall show them Our Signs upon the horizons and within themselves until it is clear to them that it is the Real (the Truth)"* (41:53).

CHAPTER 2
MICROCOSM-MACROCOSM

Spiritual warriors refer to the Signs upon the horizons as "The Book of Horizons" or macrocosm while the microcosm, the Signs within, are called "the Book of Souls." The Sign referring to these two books is in yet another Book, the Quran. The science of balance or correspondence is applied to these three books not as mathematical laws but as a kind of Abrahamic Pythogorianism.

As craftsmen, spiritual warriors are aware of the hidden sciences like numbers and geometry for these show the Signs of the Presence of God. A manifest science like ethics is also familiar to them as yet another manifestation of unity. As submitters to God's Will, they share the view of the oneness of nature:

> Know, oh Brother, that by the Universe, the sages mean the seven heavens and the earth and what is between them of all creatures. They also call it the macrocosm because it is seen that the world has one body in all its spheres, gradation of heavens, its generating elements and their production. It is also seen that it has one Soul whose power runs through all the organs of the body just like the human being who has one soul (self) which runs into all of his organs.[1]

In the study of *"the Signs upon the horizons and within themselves,"* the concept which serves as a vital link in showing the oneness of nature and the inner relationship between the human being and nature is that the human being (microcosm) is the mirror of the universe (macrocosm). Knowing the macrocosm or outer world of nature, then, becomes a means for spiritual realization just as knowing the self as the integral part of the microcosm leads to the understanding of the inner aspects of nature. Both are manifestations of God's Will seen as the processes of nature.

This concept has been expressed by poets and scholars. Jalāl al-Dīn Rūmī says:

> From the pure star-bright souls replenishment is
>   ever coming to the stars of heaven.
> Outwardly we are ruled by these stars, but our inward
>   nature has become the ruler of the skies.
> Therefore, while in form thou are the microcosm, in
>   reality, thou art the macrocosm.
> Externally the branch is the origin of the fruit;
>   intrinsically the branch came into existence
>   for the sake of the fruit.
> Had there been no hope of the fruit, would the
>   gardener have planted the tree?
> Therefore, in reality the tree is born of the fruit,
>   though it appears to be produced by the tree.[2]

Algazel puts it in one sentence: "The visible world was made to correspond to the world invisible and there is nothing in this world but is a symbol of something in that other world."[3]

Another famous Sufi poet, Maḥmūd Shabīstarī, says:

> Know the world is a mirror from head to foot.
> In every atom are a hundred blazing suns.
> If you cleave the heart of one drop of water,
> A hundred pure oceans emerge from it.
> If you examine closely each grain of sand,
> A thousand Adams may be seen in it.
> In its members, a gnat is like an elephant;
> In its qualities, a drop of rain is like the Nile.
> The heart of a barley-corn equals a hundred harvests,
> A world dwells in the heart of a millet seed.

In the wing of a gnat is the ocean of life.
In the pupil of the eye, a heaven;
What though the grain of the heart be small,
It is a station for the Lord of both worlds to dwell
    therein.[4]

One aspect of nature that receives particular emphasis by spiritual warriors is that of spiritual alchemy or the science of balance or correspondence. In this science each of the seven visible planets symbolize a corresponding metal. The operative processes of this science for spiritual warriors symbolize the struggle to realize the Presence of Reality through transforming the self.

When the "Work" begins, the self is seen as symbolized by lead which corresponds to the planet Saturn. The first change is towards tin which corresponds to the planet Jupiter. The final transmutation of lead into gold is for the spiritual warrior to transform the lead of self, developed through the nurturing process, into gold. Transformation comes from the unveiling of the Light of the nature originated by God. This Light then illuminates the spiritual aspect of the heart. Although spiritual warriors may begin the process through self-help and succeed at least in transforming from the lead to the tin of self, from the Saturn to the Jupiter of self, the final stage of actually experiencing the gold within requires the direction of a master who is the equivalent of the "Philosopher's Stone," but none of this can be done without the Presence of God.

The method of spiritual alchemy is based in cosmology rather than metaphysical or theology. The aspects of self which are made receptive to change by nature is the substance of the work. Change takes place through corresponding the external body (seen as a metal) with internal psychological states. The very objectiveness required for the transformation shows spiritual warriors that it is a path of gnosis through the language of symbols or Signs rather than love. The main Signs used in alchemy are the "hidden" sciences of numbers, geometry and letters.

At the beginning of the work, self-awareness is confused, unorganized and "heavy" much like the metal lead which corresponds to the planet Saturn. One's sense of reason is compacted, not pervious to light. Through spiritual practices like invocation, meditation and self-examination, this compactness or condensation is transformed into concentration. Through spiritual practices, the moral-seeker turns away from the outer world to the inner. The spiritual warrior becomes as a moving center descending inward into the inner self taking on an understanding of self much like the spiritual hermeneutics of the story of Moses and Khidr or Dhul Qarnayn.

The basic theory is that every metal contains a combination of sulfur and mercury which are symbolic and not to be confused with the chemical properties. For the self as lead, sulfur (reason at first confused and heavy) is heavier than mercury (the passions). These two forces, opposite and complementary, are combined with quicksilver, the breath or vital spirit, as an aspect of the Universal Soul. A balance is obtained which is the principle that measures the intensity of the Universal Soul's desire during its descent through matter or Universal Nature. The process that occurs is to transform sulfur as confused, unorganized reason into sulfur as spirit. The ash that results from the burning of sulfur and mercury, where the breath acts as the fire, is symbolized by salt. Salt, in turn, is a symbol of justice, balance.

The spiritual warrior is told through oral tradition, "Use spiritual alchemy for the knowledge of God, nature and yourself."[5] And, "The science and knowledge of all things consists in learning of the true harmony and cognizance of nature with the macrocosm and microcosm of the world and the human being, since all things originate in the One and all things in turn flow and return to One."[6]

Or, "The earth is the mirror of heaven and conversely. One is unthinkable without the other. The lights of the heavens correspond to things on the earth."[7]

Spiritual alchemy has been defined as "the voluntary action of the human being in harmony with the involuntary action of nature."[8] What nature does outside spiritual warriors, without any help from them, spiritual warriors can reproduce experimentally in their inner self."[9]

As the science of balance, spiritual alchemy is to bring the self into balance with the nature originated by God. "By balance the spiritual warrior means the essential harmony and equilibrium of things."[10]

In spiritual alchemy, for instance, the balance is between reason and the passions which is also true of psychoethics. The balance is between reason developing the positive traits held in moderation by dominating over the passions in a state of the moral reasonableness of a religiously cultured monotheist, closest to the center of self, away from the periphery of self and one's negative traits.

Just as spiritual alchemy emphasizes the balance in nature, the importance of considering the measure of things, so, too, is the concept of balance important in astrology.

In astrology the whole cycle of manifestation, temporal and spatial, is seen as an unfolding of possibilities inherent in the unique Principle which itself lies above all manifestation. All multiplicity, all diversity, is deduced from Divine Unity, especially in Islamic astrology where this perspective of revealing the relation of the cosmos to its Unique Principle is of great importance. Therefore, although astrology, in placing intermediary causes between the human being and God, is opposed to a certain aspect of the Muslim perspective, its contemplative and symbolic side conforms closely to the basic spirit of Islam which is to realize that all multiplicity comes from Unity and to seek to integrate the particular in the Universal. [11]

MICROCOSMIC SIGN OF THE PRESENCE OF GOD

Following the Sign, *"We shall show them Our Signs ....
within themselves until it is clear to them that it is the Real(the
Truth)"* (41:53), spiritual warriors turn inward. Aware of
both the manifest and the hidden sciences, practitioners of
both the Law and the Way, they seek for that which
inwardly unites self with the macrocosm and all of nature.

The description of the microcosmic Sign of the
Presence of God begins at the center. The self is described
as "a circle of unity." The circle of self begins at the center
point, itself a circle. A circle is described in the traditional
perspective as:

> .... the unitary focus of conscious awareness and the
> elusive controlling point of all forms. In traditional
> geometry—where geometry is seen in both its quantita-
> tive and qualitative aspects—the circle is considered to
> be the most excellent symbol for the origin and end of
> geometric form, a symbol of wholeness and unity. Its
> hidden center from which the outer circle was manifest-
> ed becomes as the timeless moment of the beginning of
> time 'and the dimensionless point of encompassing
> space.'[12]

The circle, in the traditional view "is the perfect expression
of justice—equal in all directions in the finite domain."[13]

The shapes used to define self in the Sign of the
Presence of God, are inseparable from the traditional concept of mathematics, particularly numbers and geometry.
Numbers and geometry are not just what they appear to
be quantitatively. They have a qualitative aspect that is as
much a part of their reality as the quantitative. Each number and geometric figure, when seen in its symbolic sense,
is an echo of Unity and a reflection of a quality contained

in principle within that Unity, which transcends all differentiation and all qualities, and yet contains them in a principal manner. The point and its relation to eternity is further delineated.

In the mind the point represents a unitary focus of conscious awareness; in the physical world it represents a focal event in a field which was previously uninterrupted...In terms of geometry it represents the center—the elusive controlling point of all forms....but also the most beautiful parent of all the polygons, both containing and underlying them. Outside the concept of time, the circle has always been regarded as a symbol of eternity, without beginning and without end, just being. As a symbol within the limits of time, or rather subject to that condition of existence, it passes around just as the active compass point returns to its first position it necessarily passes over it and in principle establishes a helix—the expression in time of the circle. The circle express 'threeness' in itself, that is, center, domain, periphery and 'fourness' in a manifest context, that is center, domain included, boundary, domain excluded.[14]

The center point of self for the spiritual warrior symbolizes first the potential, the possibility of perfecting self for it holds the possibility of mirroring everything in terms of inner meaning that the macrocosm holds. Once morally healed, the center point of self symbolizes justice, the soul at peace, the actualization of the external possibility of self or salvation.

Geometric shapes, then, are more than just technical devices. Beyond the function of a material order, they fulfill another function of even greater significance which is to remind the human self through their symbolic aspect of the spiritual principles which the traditional human being reflects on his or her own level of reality because in the traditional view, nothing is divorced from the spiritual, the inner meaning within all things.

Geometry, as the expression of the 'personality' of numbers, permits the traditional human being a further exploration into the processes of nature. The number 1 generates the point, 2 the line, and 3 the triangle. These concepts of forms, the static aspect of geometry, lead the active mind from the sensible to the intelligible, from the manifest to the hidden quality of a essential differences between a triangle and a square which measurement alone will not reveal, just as the essential difference between red and blue cannot be discovered through quantitative means alone. Expanded consciousness leads traditional man to 'seek knowledge unto China,' to copy of 'nature in her mode of operation,' not in her manifested form. The triangle and the square are not merely shapes; essentially they incorporate a reality the understanding of which through *taw''il* leads man to the world of similitudes and ultimately to the Truth.[15]

There are two triangular shapes in the Sign of the Presence of God. According to the traditional view, nature provides the self with three functions which can be perfected through free-will and reason, in effect, providing human beings with the ability to surmount nature. One triangular form divides the self at center point into three segments of 120 degrees each symbolizing the threefold division of the self. They are cognition, attraction to pleasure (affect) and avoidance of harm (behavior). Each segment of this triangular form then divides into three segments of 40 degrees each. $3 \times 3 = 9$.

The other triangle clusters around the center point symbolizing the three positive traits of wisdom, temperance and courage. When taken as three points along with the nine points of the 40 degree divisions of the threefold segment, each segment contains four points. $3 \times 4 = 12$.

Three as the threefold division of the self symbolizes the three basic movements of the spirit—ascending, descending, and horizontal. This can be further understood in terms of the traditional system of colors.

Three as number and as triangle in geometry reflects the fundamental conception of spirit, soul and body which makes up all of creation. Viewed alternatively as the three motions of the spirit, it evokes the acts of descent, ascent, and horizontal expansion which exhibit, respectively, passive, active and neutral qualities.

White is the integration of all colors, pure and unstained. In its unmanifested state it is the color of Pure Light before individualization, before the One became the many. Light, symbolically viewed as white, descends from the sun and symbolizes Unity.

As it is through white that color is made manifest, so through black it remains hidden, "hidden by its very brightness." Black is "a bright light in a dark day," as only through this luminous black can one find the hidden aspects of the Divine. This perception comes through the black of the pupil which, as the center of the eye, is symbolically the veil to both internal and external vision. Black is the annihilation of self, prerequisite to reintegration. It is the cloak of the Kabah, the mystery of Being, the light of Majesty, and the color of the Divine.

Sandalwood is the color of earth, void of color. It is the neutral based upon which nature (the system of four colors) and the polar qualities of black and white act.[16]

Three also symbolizes the threefold division of the self: intellectual, emotional and volitional or thinking, feeling and actions. Other terms used for the threefold division are cognition, perception and motivation or reason, attraction to pleasure and avoidance of harm/pain.

A most basic instinctive level in relation to the nature originated by God (*fiṭrat Allāh*) three relates to first, the natural instinct to preserve the eternal possibility of self (cognition, reason, the spirit, the intellect, wisdom both theoretical and practical), second, the natural instinct to preserve the individual (avoidance of harm/pain, defensive aspects of self), and third, the natural instinct to preserve the species (attraction to pleasure).

Biologically three symbolizes three sources of energy: liver (gut), heart, and brain. These three sources of energy can also be called affect (A), behavior (B), and cognition (C) which are the symbols used in the Sign throughout this handbook.

The same three segments are often combined and expressed in terms of reason vs. the passions, reason symbolized by (C) and the passions by (A) and (B). A and B are also called the animal self or *nafs ammārah* while C is referred to as the *nafs lawwāmah* or blaming, reproaching self. The center symbolizes the self at peace (*nafs muṭma'innah*).

Three also symbolizes harmony. It is the first odd number and 1/3 of all numbers are counted by it. In the microcosm it is symbolized by two extremities and a middle.

The threefold division of the circle, (A), (B) and (C) extends to the edges of the outer circle as the underlying psychological structure of self neutral at the psychological level to moral balance or imbalance. Each of these three segments, however, also represent a moral imbalance based on the psychological aspect of self. The moral imbalance in either of the three segments may be in terms of quantity or quality. If the imbalance is in terms of quantity it may be either an underdevelopment of the moral trait symbolized by that segment or an overdevelopment. In terms of quality, an imbalance is symbolized by underdevelopment. That is, the moral trait never developed.

Each of the three segments of the other circle, then, has three possibilities of moral imbalance which are delineated in the next section. In the top segment, symbolizing the brain and referred to as cognition (C), overdevelopment of the natural system of cognition can be represented as (+) which represents the moral imbalance of hypocrisy (*nifāq*) Underdevelopment is the ability to reason can be represented by (-) which represents multitheism (*shirk*), worshipping more gods than there are for the spiritual warrior. Undevelopment represented by (o) is to show ingratitude and disbelief in the One God (*kufr*), a moral state lacking in wisdom (faith in the One God) in terms of quality.

Segment (B) symbolizes behavior. It is located in the heart and referred to as avoidance of harm/pain, preservation of the individual or an aspect of "the passions." Overdevelopment of avoidance of harm/pain is represented as the moral imbalance of recklessness arising out of inappropriate anger. Underdevelopment is a state of cowardice while undevelopment (o) is fear of anything other than God, a state of moral imbalance lacking in the positive moral trait of courage (trust in God).

Segment (A) symbolizes affect. It is located in the liver (gut). Known as the attraction to pleasure function to preserve the species, it is the center of feelings as an aspect of "the passions." Overdevelopment is manifested as greed and inappropriate lust as well as the desire for worldly things. Underdevelopment is expressed as apathy or the lack of self-esteem and self-identity. Undevelopment is symbolized by envy, a state of moral imbalance lacking in the quality of the positive trait of temperance (charity towards others).

The outer circle is now complete with nine points (3x3) on the circumference. As an added distinction, those three qualities known as undevelopment of a positive trait in terms of quality are so far removed from a sense of balance and centeredness that they fall just outside the circle.

The Quran refers to the nine negative traits we will be describing below. The Sign says:

> *In the city there were nine persons who did corruption in*
> *the land. They said to each other, "Swear you, one to another,*
> *by God, 'We will attack him and his family by night.' Then*
> *we will tell his protector, 'We were not witnesses of the*
> *destruction of his family and assuredly we are truthful men.'"*
> *They plotted and planned but We too planned while they were*
> *not aware. Behold how was the end of their plan for We*
> *destroyed them and their people all together. Those are their*
> *houses all fallen down because of the evil they committed.*
> *Surely in this is a Sign for a people who have knowledge of the*
> *inner self. And We delivered those who believed and those*
> *who had piety* (27:48-83).

According to spiritual hermeneutics, the Signs say: <u>In the city</u> of the body, <u>there were nine persons</u>, nine negative traits <u>who did corruption in the land</u>, who corrupted the moral balance of the body. These nine negative traits, waged a relentless war against justice [that is, against moral healing and being balanced and centered in self, against regaining the moral reasonableness of a religiously cultured monotheist].

<u>They</u>, these nine negative traits, <u>said to each other,</u> "<u>Swear you, one to another, by God, 'We will attack him,'</u> the heart, '<u>and his family,'</u> his physical and psychic forces, '<u>by night,'</u> when the heart is in a state of heedlessness, forgetfulness. "<u>Then we will tell his protector</u>," the spirit, the intellect, reason, "<u>We were not witnesses of the destruction of his family and assuredly we are truthful men</u>." That is, the nine negative traits ban together to attack the heart so that it becomes so confused that it turns away from its struggle for moral balance. The negative aspects of self have no conscience so they are able to lie to reason with ease. <u>They</u>, the nine negative traits, <u>plotted and planned but We too planned while they were not aware</u>. That is, Divine Grace planned and guided the heart secretly towards moral balance without the nine negative traits

knowing about it. "Behold," says the Quran, "how was the end of their plan," that is, the plan of the nine negative traits to upset the moral balance of the heart," for We destroyed them and their people all together." That is, through Divine intervention, the heart is able at one time, in one moment, to destroy the nine negative traits and morally heal. Those are their houses, that is, their places within the self, all fallen down, illuminated and destroyed because of the evil they, the nine negative traits, committed. Surely in this is a Sign, of "the Presence of God," for a people who have knowledge of the inner self. And We delivered those who believed and those who had piety, that is, spiritual warriors (27:48-53).

Nature provides the heart with four positive traits as aspects of that nature originated by God through which to attain moral balance. They are symbolized by wisdom (belief in the One God), courage (trust in the One God), temperance (charity towards others) and justice (putting Reality in Its proper place), the latter arising out of the center which formed the circle of self when the other three positive traits are held in moderation.

Just as we have seen the system of three colors, there is a system of four, together forming the system of seven colors.

Four as number and as square in geometry reflects the conceptual configuration of Universal Soul manifested as the active qualities of nature (hot, cold, wet, dry) and the passive qualities of matter (fire, water, air, and earth)....

In vision, the primary colors are red, yellow, green and blue. These four colors correspond to the four qualities of Universal Nature and to the four elements of matter. Nature, the active agent towards matter, initiates the temporal creative process and determines the rhythms of the inner and the outer aspects of all being. Through the system of the four colors, man establishes sensible correspondences with the various aspects of this inherent energy of nature that is continuously in search of a state of equilibrium analogous to its primordial state of order.

Red develops an association with fire, exhibiting the paired natural qualities of heat and dryness. It expresses the vital spirit—active, expansive and insoluble. Cyclically, it is morning, spring, and childhood. The complement of red is green, which exhibits the opposite qualities of coldness and humidity. Green characterizes water, the superior soul, passive, contractive, and soluble qualities. Cyclically, it is evening, fall, and maturity. Yellow is air, hot and wet. Its qualities are contemplative, active, expansive, and soluble. It stands for noon, summer, and youth. It complements blue, which represents earth, cold and dry. The inferior soul, passive, contractive, and insoluble are its qualities, while symbolically it represents the end of the cycles, for it is night, winter, and old age. Viewed as a movement through the four quadrants of a circle, the descending and ascending motions of these colors describe a full circle: the end of one cycle only signals the beginning of another.[17]

Four is manifested everywhere in nature as stability and the first square number. Four also symbolizes expansion, fixation, contraction, and solution, terms used in spiritual alchemy and the four stages of energy: solid, liquid, gas, and radiation.

> God has made it such that the majority of things of Nature are grouped in four such as the four physical natures which are hot, cold, wet, and dry; the four elements which are fire, air, water and earth; the four humors which are blood, phlegm, yellow bile and black bile.....[18]

and the four positive traits of wisdom, courage, temperance and justice.

To be balanced and centered means that the four positive traits are balanced in terms of the natural qualities of the elements.

Hot and dry shows coherence and cohesion, subtlety and ascending motion. Its form is like the upright stance of the *alif* or first letter of the Arabic alphabet or the Pen or the tall flame or the cypress. These forms symbolize the tendency of the parts of a substance to move towards one center, one area of being. It is blood of the four humors.

Hot and wet refers to swelling, expansion, the opposite effects of dryness. Hot here also requires an ascending motions, symbolized by a pine-cone or the triangle pointing upwards. It is yellow bile of the four humors.

Cold and wet manifests expansion because of humidity while coldness demands descending movement and the absence of all spontaneous upward movement. It revolves upon itself and its form is spherical, the most corpulent of all forms. It lacks compactness and cohesion while its constitutent parts tend toward dispersion and thus towards transparency. It is phlegm of the humors.

Cold and dry refers to the compactness and cohesion of the parts while the coldness demands movement downwards. Its form is a toothed form with angles and dents. It is black bile in the humors.[19]

Four, then, symbolizes harmony in nature, so here, the self is at rest, at peace, manifesting the "self at peace" (*nafs mutma'innah*). The heart has been turned towards its spiritual aspect. The spiritual aspect of the heart is said to be unveiled by the Light of the nature originated by God and it is now able to relate to nature and other human beings as a trustee of the manifestation of a socioethics based in theoethics.

The Sign of the heart is now complete, symbolizing the illumination of the inner Light. With the illumination of the inner Light symbolically located at the center of self, spiritual warriors have retraced their steps back to their nature originated by God. This nature is what is called religion and for spiritual warriors it is the belief in the One God, the Creator of the macrocosm and the microcosm. Having illuminated the inner Light also means to spiritual warriors that they are in control of the fluctuations of their heart. This control allows them to turn it towards the spiritual and away from the material because they have succeeded in morally healing themselves. Their success means that reason has been victorious in its struggles with the passions for the attention of the heart.

The heart, the center point, symbolizes the morally healed spiritual warrior centered in justice. To be centered in justice means the self holds positive traits of wisdom, courage and temperance in moderation. It means that reason (cognition, the intellect, the spirit) dominates over the passions. It means that the self has managed to balance the four elements of earth, air, fire and water in their universal qualities of hot, cold, moist and dry in balance.

It consists of a center point (justice, piety, putting Reality in Its place, to manifest the moral reasonableness of a religiously cultured monotheist, the *nafs muṭma'innah*) surrounded by a circle of three equal segments (the three energy sources of self) within which is an equilateral triangle, the three points of which symbolize courage (3*), temperance (6*) and wisdom (9*) with justice in the center.

> ...the minimal expression of an area and the simplest figure to which all other polygons can be reduced. It is also symbolic of the minimal needs of consciousness (i.e. knower, known and the act of knowing).[20]

One-third of the equilateral triangle touches each of the three segments of the circle of unity. This equilateral triangle is clustered around the center—as close to the center as possible, the center being the source of Light.

The Sign then begins to take further shape symbolic of the nurturing process. The center point having formed the outer circle, its threefold division and equilateral triangle we have seen are symbolic of the morally balanced person. The outer circle encompasses a distance between the heart and the nurtured self. The concept of distance is important because the negative traits assumed through the nurturing process are mentioned as being on the periphery, the farthest distance possible from the center, the source of Light. The outer circle symbolizes the state of ignorance of Reality. Looking from the center outwards, it is a subjective view we have here and not an objective one. This furthers the practice of self-examination.

Three plus four equals seven, the next significant number of the unfolding of the Sign of the Presence of God. Seven is the first complete number, odd, square, exceeding and perfect. It symbolizes the active powers within the microcosm (attraction, sustenance, digestion, repulsion, nutrition, growth, and formation).

The Divine Names and Qualities form a hierarchy which corresponds to the perfections of Divine Essence. While the Names and Qualities are infinite, their sources are seven: Life, Knowledge, Power, Will, Speech, Hearing and Sight. These Qualities form the seven Divine Names of perfection, namely, the Living, the Knowing, the Powerful, the Willing, the Speaking, the Hearing, and the Seeing.[21]

A traditional teaching in spiritual chivalry is that there are two kinds of pilgrimages: one is the pilgrimage of the believers to the Kabah in Makkah and the other is the pilgrimage of the spiritual warrior and that is the desire for the Presence of the Divine Friend. Just as there is the outward Kabah to which spiritual warriors orient their prayers, so there is an inner Kabah which embraces the Throne of God according to the Divine Tradition, "My heavens and My earth do not embrace Me but the heart of My believing servant does embrace Me."

The Kabah (cube) is an extension of 4:

>According to the Euclidean generation of geometry through lines, 4 as a static form becomes the square; extended and dynamic, it becomes the cross. The square as 4, or the cube as 6, is the most arrested and inactive of shapes. It represents the most externalized and fixed aspects of creation. The cube is therefore regarded as the symbol of earth in the macroscale and man in the microscale. The 'cube of man' is a symbolic representation of his manifested characteristics—the coordinate system of the six directions—which he shares with the earth and the heavens. The hexahedron then symbolizes the last manifestation—in the planets, earth, and among matter, man. It is the supreme temporal symbol of Islam, as Kabah means cube.[22]

The external Kabah being a center is the place around which believers circumambulate seven times.

>The Kabah is an outward symbol in this material world of that Presence not seen by the eye, which dwells within the Divine world, just as the body is an outward symbol of this visible phenomenal world, of the heart, which cannot be seen by the eye, for it belongs to the world of the Unseen, and this material, visible world is a means of ascent to the invisible, spiritual world for him to whom God has opened the door.[23]

This Kabah has an inner correspondence as does the circumambulation since every center is somehow connected to every other and circumambulation is associated with center. *"Everyone has a part of heaven towards which he orients himself"* (2:148); *"Whichever way you turn, there is the Presence of God"* (2:115)

It is said in the Traditions that when God announced to the angels that He would be creating a vicegerent on earth, the angels asked, *"What! will You set therein one who will do corruption there and shed blood while We proclaim Your praise and call you Holy?"* He said, *"Clearly I know what you know not."* (2:30)

According to a Tradition, with this response, the angels sense that the Divine Light was being veiled from them. They then seek refuge near the Throne where seventy thousand angels appear each day. They circumambulate the Throne for seven days, seven symbolizing the seven millenia of the Prophets.

God then commands the angels to descend to earth and build a Kabah which would be the image of the Kabah in the world of the Universal Soul. This is the Kabah around which Prophet Adam and his children circumambulated seven times in imitation of the angels. During the time of Prophet Noah, the Kabah is destroyed in the flood or said to have been removed to the fourth heaven by the angels because human beings had become unworthy of seeing it.

Centuries later, Prophet Abraham, the spiritual exile and founder of spiritual chivalry, rebuilds the Kabah on the foundations of the one which had disappeared. As it is built upon the original foundations, "This is how the Abrahamic pilgrim," the spiritual warrior, "in performing the external rituals," around the Kabah, "knows that his true pilgrimage is being accomplished around the invisible Kabah" within the spiritual world.[24] To approach the Divine Presence is to circumambulate the Kabah seven times in an attempt to seek refuge in its enclosure, its center symbolizing the center of self. It is in this sense that the Kabah symbolizes the Throne and the Throne, as we have seen, "...*was upon the Waters*" (11:7). Nothing in the universe can embrace the Throne but the heart of the believer when it turns towards "the Presence of God."

The symbolic significance of seven is confirmed by spiritual warriors when they divide seven by the six numbers which precede it beginning with one, unity. The result is a recurring decimal which appears six times in different order but in no case does the first six decimals contain 3's, 6's or 9's. When the numbers of the decimal obtained—1, 4, 2, 8, 5, 7— are drawn connecting the numbers on the circumference of the outer circle into nine parts, a line called the line of change or movement appears indicating the path of moral healing moving backwards through the circle from (C) to (B) to (B) to (C) to (A) to (A) and back to (C). Each of the recurring decimals of dividing unity gives a different pattern as will be explained.

It is significant that this recurring decimal gives no 3's, 6's, or 9's. 3, 6 and 9 symbolized with an asterisk are the positive traits of courage (3*), temperance (6*) and wisdom (9*). With the (o) sign they symbolize the lack of quality of the segment's characteristics and are referred to as undeveloped. In terms of numbers, 1 divided by 3 gives a recurring decimal of .333 while 1 divided by 6 gives another recurring decimal of .666. Nine divided by 1 gives 1, unity, oneness.

Nine is yet another important number for the spiritual warrior. The Quran says that when God creates He only says "'Be!' *and it is*" (6:73). Be in Arabic is *kun*. The root of this verb is *kwn*:

> .....*kāf, wāw, nūn*. When these three letters are multiplied by the three letters which compose, respectively, the name of each, the resulting figure is nine. It is this number that regulates the structure of being with regard to both the esoteric and the exoteric, the visible world or the world of the Universal Soul.[25]

The Divine Intellect moves in "threeness," horizontal, descending and ascending. The equilateral triangle expresses the number 3. Doubling 3, inverting the equilateral triangle upon itself, becomes 6 or the hexagram. Three times itself is 9 whereby each of the three equilateral triangles reflect the symmetry of the other, showing multiplicity in unity.

Nine is further described in traditional arithmetic:

Number admits nothing beyond the ennead, but rather everything circles around within it. This is clear from the so-called recurrences: there is natural progression up to it, but after it there is repetition. For 10 becomes a monad by the subtraction of one elementary quantity.... so that it is by no means possible for there to subsist any number beyond the nine elementary numbers. Hence they called it 'ocean' and 'horizon', because it encompasses both of these locations and has them within itself....

The ennead is the first square based on an odd number. It ... is called 'that which brings completion', and it completes nine-month children; moreover it is called 'perfect', because it arises out of 3, which is a perfect number. The heavenly spheres revolve around the Earth, which is ninth....[26]

Nine is symbolized in the Quran by the 9 miracles Prophet Moses used against Pharaoh and his magicians. The nine miracles include: the Rod,[27] the Radiant Hand,[28] Famine,[29] Short crops,[30] Epidemics among men and beasts, Locusts, Lice, Frogs, and water turning to blood.[31] In regard to the rod, spiritual hermeneutics of the verse say:

The Rod of Moses symbolizes the animal self (the passions) of Moses which he leaned on every step he took. He used the animal self to guide his animalistic forces which are natural to the human being. He also used the animal self to guide his social behavior and to demonstrate the positive traits and praiseworthy habits as drawn from the tree of the intellect. For that reason, the animal self of Moses was well directed because of the good manners he imposed on it and his training of it. The animal self was subjected to His actions, obedient to His commands, reticent towards animalistic behavior because he was in control of it.

The animal self is like the rod. When you throw it (the animal self) down in the face of opponents, it becomes like the serpent that will swallow their falsehood and lies. The opponents to the self—negative traits—forge lies, create suspicion and doubt.

By his Radiant Hand, Moses demonstrated his overwhelming power to enthrall Pharaoh's magicians and to reveal the manifestation of the light of the truth of his claim (the One he is calling them to).[32]

The microcosmic Sign of the Presence of God, then, is composed of numbers and geometry understood in the sense of Abrahamic Pythagoreanism. In terms of numbers, it consists of numbers 1-9 which each has its particular inner correspondence as we have seen. In terms of geometry, it consists of center point, circumference, threefold division of the circle into 120 degree segments, ninefold division of the circle in 40 degree segments and an equilateral triangle, the center of which is the same center of self through which the Sign unfolded.

In terms of correspondences to other aspects of nature, the center once illuminated by the Light of nature originated by God becomes known as "the Throne" and "the Kabah," the place which is prepared to sense the Presence of God.

As to moral balance, the outer circle symbolizes the state of ignorance of Reality (*jahl*) while the center point surrounded by the equilateral triangle symbolizes the state of the moral reasonableness of a religiously cultured monotheist (*ḥilm*).

MACROCOSMIC SIGN OF THE PRESENCE OF GOD

Returning to the Sign, *"We shall show them Our Signs upon the horizons,"* spiritual warriors turn outward to find the macrocosmic correspondence of the Sign of the Presence of God. One of the most significant natural phenomenon to the followers of the Way are the 12 constellations, Zodiac or fixed stars. God swears an oath by them in the Quran, *"By the sky displaying the Zodiacal Signs..."* (85:1). The Zodiac for the spiritual warrior indicate periods of time and direction in space.

The indication of periods of time and directions in space occurs in pattern form as intervals around the perimeter of this primal circle. For instance, the face of a clock with its twelve hourly divisions exemplifies the measuring of the passage of time with precision, whereas if one should join these same intervals on the clock-face with straight lines, one would describe a twelve-sided shape—a dodecagon. Both can be taken as expressions of the archetype twelve, and in cosmology they are united temporally and spatially in one complete annual cycle of our planet: the twelve zodiacal constellations give us both a directional guide and specific periods of time by which to measure the whole year.[33]

The twelve Signs contain the four elements and their universal qualities which are then filtered down through the planets to the moon and then to the earth. They also move in the way the spirit moves—ascending, descending, and horizontal. Ibn al-'Arabī refers each to a Quranic Sign, as well.

♈	Aries:	"those who repel evil" (37:2)
♉	Taurus:	"those who proclaim God's Message" (37:3)
♊	Gemini:	"those who distribute by Command" (51:4)
♋	Cancer:	"those who are sent forth (like the winds)" (77:1)
♌	Leo:	"those who disperse one after another to the benefit of humanity" (77:1)
♍	Virgo:	"those who seize the wrongdoers" (79:1)
♎	Libra:	"those who gently extract (the blessed)" (79:2)
♏	Scorpio:	"those who precede, press forward" (79:4)
♐	Sagittarius:	"those who guide along (on errands of mercy)" (79:3)
♑	Capricorn:	"those who spread abroad a Message" (77:5)
♒	Aquarius:	"those who arrange the Commands of their Lord" (79:5)
♓	Pisces:	"those who arrange themselves in ranks" (37:1)[34]

From another perspective they are said to be veils which hide "the Face" or "Presence" of God because above the heavens of the fixed stars is the Throne of God which was upon the Waters, *"and His Throne was upon the Waters"* (11:7).

Here we note that the first being created in the higher universe, according to traditional cosmology, was Light which contains all light. The Light of Lights is described in spiritual chivalry as the Throne, the Intellect. First in the lower world was primordial water—not one of the four elements. The water is also known as the Throne. The Throne rests on the Water. This relationship is consolidated by the function of the twelve constellations. We will have occasion to recall this later.

The twelve Signs are described as having spiritual

forces which change the nature of bodies submitted to their influence. This is done through a natural philosophy that is based in the four natures or qualities and the four elements.

The second major emphasis in the heavens for traditional cosmology is the presence of the seven planets visible to the naked eye, namely, Saturn, Jupiter, Mars, the Sun, Venus, Mercury and the Moon.

The heaven of the fixed stars is called the heaven of the stations because the movement of the planets project themselves upon it. The seven planets, which represent the cosmic intermediaries between the immutable world of the archetypes and the earthly center, actualize, by their combined rhythms and the reciprocal positions which ensure, the spatial relations virtually contained in the indefinite sphere of the sky-limit, the sphere being no other than the totality of the directions of the space and hence, the image of the universe.[35]

The twelve Signs of the Zodiac and the seven visible planets are described symbolically as revolving in circular form. This form is particularly important in traditional geometry as we have seen. Here, for instance, when the circle is divided into sixty equidistant intervals:

We find the number of divisions which links by multiplication the perfect number six with the other perfect number, ten. We see that this division of sixty, while in a cosmological sense relating to a sixty year cycle, also belongs to a traditional division of time and space—sixty seconds and sixty minutes. This number of divisions of the circle is the smallest which enable the basic geometric polygons to co-ordinate—the equilateral triangle, the square, the pentagon and the hexagon. In each case the points of the polygon sit within the regular intervals which are shown subdivided into twelve groups of five. As we have seen, all these shapes are primary, both geometrically in terms of the laws of space division and as representatives of numerical archetypes.[36]

This cycle of sixty years then corresponds to time (*zaman*). When we look to the symbolism of letters where only the consonants are counted, the three consonants *z*, *m*, and *n* are the exact same three as the word for balance, *mizan*. Again, an important correspondence for the spiritual warrior. The circle of the twelve Signs of the Zodiac and the seven visible planets is a symbol of balance at the macrocosmic level.

The connection of time and balance is found in many Signs of the Quran. Ibn al-'Arabī introduces them as follows:

> The prophet has said: I and the final hour are like these two (fingers). And God himself has said: *We will establish the balance in equilibrium on the day of Resurrection* (21:47). And we are told: *Weigh justly, and do not falsify the balance* (55:9). And again: *He has raised the Heavens and established the balance* (55:7). Thus, by means of the balance, God has revealed in each heaven the function of that heaven (41:12). And by means of the balance He has distributed proportionately over the earth the foods that the earth produces (41:10). And God Most High has set up a balance in the universe for each thing: a spiritual balance and a material balance. The balance never errs. In this way the Balance [the Libra] enters into speech and into all the arts whose object is perceived by the senses. In the same way, it enters into Ideas, for the primary origin of terrestrial bodies and celestial bodies, and of the Ideas which they support, is found in the law of the Balance. Similarly, the existence of time and of that which is above time proceeds from the Divine Balance to which the Name the Wise (*hakīm*)

aspires, and which is made manifest by the equitable Judge. After the Balance (Libra), Scorpio is manifested together with the *res divina* which God has placed in it. Then come Sagittarius, Capricorn, and so on.[37]

The conclusion reached by Ibn al-'Arabī is that the beginning and the end of time relate to the zodiacal sign of Libra (Balance). "Every cycle of time ends in the Balance."[38] It is from the Sign of Libra that all other Signs are manifested because it is the Sign of the harmony of things and of divine equity, the notion of equilibrium and balance. It is balance which gives time its cyclical form.

The balance returns to equilibrium at the end of the cycle, and this equilibrium is the return of time to the starting point which then becomes once more the starting point of a new cycle. We said at the outset that the science of the Balance is the very foundation of the correspondences between the worlds: without the idea of the balance, there can be no worlds in correspondence with each other. The correspondences established ...would be impossible if the only image they possessed was of time as rectilinear and unlimited, like that of present-day evolutionism. Thanks to the Balance, it is possible to set in correspondence the figures which are found in every cycle, for they are then seen to be homologous.[39]

Seven corresponds with the seven visible planets and with the seven subtle centers or seven Prophets of our being. These seven Prophets are those who brought the Divine Law, namely, Adam, Noah, Abraham, Moses, David, Jesus and Muhammad.

The two planets which are of particular significance to us here are that of Saturn and Jupiter. Saturn in the macrocosm corresponds to Prophet Abraham and Jupiter to Moses. Prophet Abraham, as we have seen, was the founder of spiritual chivalry and Prophet Moses was given nine miracles to use against Pharaoh. *"To Moses We did give Nine Clear Signs..."* (17:101). Pharaoh symbolizes the idol/ego within.

The seven visible planets also correspond to seven of the Most Beautiful Names of God. In this schema, Saturn corresponds to Lord (*rabb*) and that of Jupiter to the Knower (*'alim*).

> The sky of Saturn is attributed to the Divine Name *ar-Rabb*, 'the Lord', the meaning of which implies a reciprocal relationship, because a being has no quality of lordship except in relation to a servant, and the servant is not thus a servant except in relation to a lord. For the created being, this relationship has a necessary and unalterable character whereas the other divine qualities can in some ways vary in color according to the individual. The sky of Jupiter is the complement of the Divine Name *al-'alim*, 'the Knower'.[40]

Here the famous Tradition comes to mind, "He who knows himself, knows His Lord." That is, the knowing of self in order to know one's Lord comes in the conjunction of the sky of Saturn and that of Jupiter.

In the cosmological schema of the phrase, "In the Name of Allah, the Merciful, the Compassionate," which every chapter but one begins with in the Quran, Saturn and Jupiter fall between the two l's of Allah.[41] In the science of numbers, the 3x3 magic square corresponds to Saturn, similar to the 3x3 negative traits of the outer circle of the microcosmic Sign of the Presence of God, while the 4x4 magic square to Jupiter.[42] Together 3 x 4 = 12. Again, 3 + 4 = 7.

As may have been surmised to this point, Saturn and Jupiter form the macrocosmic Sign of the Presence of God in a major astrological phenomenon which occurs every sixty years. The following study of the movement of these two planets is taken from 1940-2000 AD.[43]

Figure 1 shows the trigonal relationship in the circle of the Zodiac or "fixed stars" caused by the conjunction of Saturn and Jupiter in 1940, 1960 and 1980. This forms what is called the great trigon when they are simultaneously in the same Sign of the Zodiac every twenty years. In 1940, they are together in Taurus; in 1960, in Capricorn; and in 1980, in Virgo. These three Signs are the earth Signs—cold and dry.

Figure 2 shows Saturn and Jupiter in a time relationship of 120 degrees from each other. Saturn is in Leo and Jupiter is in Sagittarius in 1947. Saturn is in Aries and Jupiter is in Leo in 1967 and in 1987, Saturn is in Sagittarius and Jupiter is in Aries. Connecting these time relationships gives a second equilateral triangular pattern and these are the Signs of fire, hot and dry.

Figure 3 shows that in 1941, both Saturn and Jupiter were in Gemini; in 1961 both were in Aquarius; and in 1981, both were in Libra. One could read this equilateral triangle in another way, as well, in another twenty year pattern. In 1953, Saturn was in Libra and Jupiter was in Gemini; in 1973, Saturn was in Gemini and Jupiter was in Aquarius; in 1993, Saturn was in Aquarius and Jupiter was in Libra. Connecting these 120 degree time relationships gives a third equilateral triangular pattern and these are the Signs of air—hot and moist.

Figure 4 shows the three equilateral triangles superimposed on each other. This pattern occurs every sixty years. The figure shows the connection between the sixty year cycle and a nine-pointed star or "the triangular relationships that relate symmetrically in a nine-fold pattern."[44]

Figure 5 shows the pattern that Jupiter makes during each sixty year cycle in relationship to Saturn. The pattern is based on a seven year interval. In 1940, Jupiter is in Taurus; in 1947, in Sagittarius; in 1954, in Gemini; in 1961, in Capricorn; in 1968, in Leo; in 1974, in Aquarius; in 1980, in Virgo; in 1987, in Aries; in 1993, in Libra. Jupiter, we see, has moved backwards in trigonal relationship to Saturn in a pattern of a nine-pointed star, each point being seven years from the next. The nine-pointed star is one of dynamic geometry.

Figure 6 shows the pattern of Saturn in the same sixty year cycle. It moves in a slower pattern than Jupiter. In 1940, it was in Taurus; in 1949, it was in Leo; in 1953, it was in Libra; in 1961, in Capricorn; in 1968, in Aries; in 1974, in Gemini; in 1980, in Virgo; in 1987, in Sagittarius; in 1993, in Aquarius. Saturn forms the pattern of a static nine-pointed star skipping one Sign at each edge as it moves through the nine divisions of the circle.

Saturn and Jupiter, then, every sixty years form a nine-pointed star pattern in intervals of seven years. It is interesting to note that in the same sixty year period, Saturn and Jupiter also form the "Seal of Solomon" or a six-pointed star when they are in 180 degrees from each other three times during the sixty year period (Figure 7). These occur in 1951, 1971 and 1991.

Where they are opposite to each other at 180 degrees, not being included in the nine point unfolding, they are in the three water Signs of Pisces, Scorpio and Cancer, cold and wet in elemental qualities (Figure 8). The nine point forms created by Saturn and Jupiter, rest, in a sense, upon the water as the symbol of the Throne of God located in the heavens beyond Saturn recalling the Sign, "And His Throne was upon the Waters," (11:7).

This is the place which is referred to by Rūmī as the stage of walāyah (friend of God).

> The friends of God have, in addition to these known heavens, seen other heavens for they no longer esteem these known heavens which seem to them too paltry. They have transcended them and left them

behind. And how can it surprise us that one of us men should be enabled to pass beyond Saturn?[45]

Another mystic poet, Farīd al-Dīn Aṭṭār said, "If this knot is united to you, your dwelling will be the head of Saturn."[46] The ascent beyond Saturn becomes a return 'home' for the Sufi.

Ibn al-'Arabī quotes the sacred Tradition of the Messenger, "My heavens and My earth embrace Me not but the heart of My believing servant does embrace Me." To embrace God means to have knowledge of God and this knowledge in the case of spiritual chivalry means experiential knowledge. This experiential knowledge leads to the sensing of the Presence of God in all that one does, the presence of Divine Grace, Divine Spirit. In this state, the heart becomes the Throne of God as Ibn al-'Arabī describes it resting on the three-fold division of the self.

The numbers 3, 6 and 9 on the circumference of the circle as they relate to the Zodiac in astrological symbolism are cold and dry while the numbers 1, 4, 2, 8, 5, and 7 on the circumference of the circle relate to the Zodiacal Signs that are hot and wet or dry relating the Sign of the Presence of God to traditional medicine where correspondence exists between illnesses and the four qualities of hot, cold, wet and dry. With that in mind 3, 6, and 9 in terms of the Zodiac are symbolic of cold/dry and 1, 4, 2, 8, 5, and 7 are hot/wet, dry.

Just as *"His Throne was upon the Waters,"* as the Sign says referring to the macrocosm, so, too, there is a significant correspondence in the microcosm. The threefold division of the self corresponds to the points where Saturn and Jupiter are 180 degrees from each other in the Signs of Pisces, Scorpio and Cancer which are the Signs of water, cold and wet. Cold and wet at the microcosmic level are the constituents of clay. A Sign says, *"We created the human being out of an extraction of clay"* (23:12). The correspondence extends even further. Just as the heavenly *"Throne was upon the Waters,"* (11:7), so, too, the earthly throne, the heart of the believer, sits upon the waters of the threefold division of the self. These three water Signs are then not included in the Sign of the Presence of God as numbers but as geometric divisions. This is how the twelve becomes the nine.

The numbers of the line of change, 7 divided by the numbers of 1 to 6 are then, symbolic of the elemental quality of heat. Moral healing comes through what is considered to be hot—cohesion, coherence, subtlety and ascending motion. "This is the result of the tendencies of a substance's constitutive parts to move towards one center, one area of being."[47]

The Sign of the Presence of God, then, corresponds to the macrocosm and the conjunctions of the planetary spheres of Saturn and Jupiter which lie just below the Throne in traditional cosmology. We have understood the nature aspect of self-center point, circle, threefold division, equilateral triangle and four positive traits and its correspondence to the Throne of God. We have developed the outer circle symbolizing the nurturing process and the nine points as well as the line of movement from segment to segment backwards through the outer circle to effect moral healing.

The heart is also known as the Kabah, cube, the Kabah of the self. When the points are connected in each of the three segments with the positive trait of that segment, three parallelograms are formed and again 3 x 4 = 12 and the Sign has yet another correspondence with the macrocosm which form the top and sides of a cube.

Correspondence of the functional relationships between the twelve Signs of the Zodiac and the twelve points of the Sign of the Presence of God reflect the concept that everything in the lower world is a projection and image of something in the higher world. From the macro-cosmic heavens emanate energies which are shared between the Signs of the Zodiac and the Sign of the Presence of God. That is, God's Presence through *"Signs upon the horizons and within themselves"* (41:53). For the spiritual warrior, it has become clear that they are *"the Real (the Truth)"* (41:53).

Considering the use of numbers and geometry in their symbolic and qualitative aspect, the spiritual warrior now has a Sign by which to further effect self-examination. It is a growth oriented, continuous process and when done through the Sign of the Presence of God, the spiritual warrior has greater potential to morally heal, to arise out of the state of ignorance of Reality to the moral reasonableness of a religiously cultured monotheist.

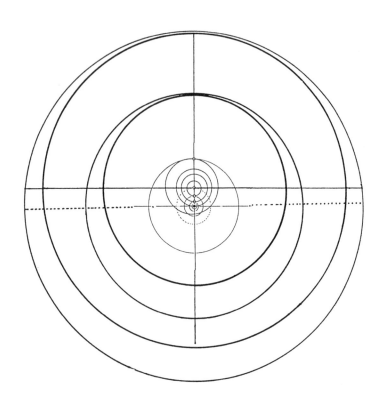

**PSYCHOLOGICAL MODEL OF THE
MACROCOSM-MICROCOSM CORRESPONDENCE**

This diagram shows a section through the solar system where the orbits of the planets are drawn symbolically in concentric circles. The diagram represents "the traditional psychological model [of the universe] and a direct perceptual response to man's actual experience of the universe." See Keith Critchlow, *Islamic Patterns*, p. 152 for a full discussion.

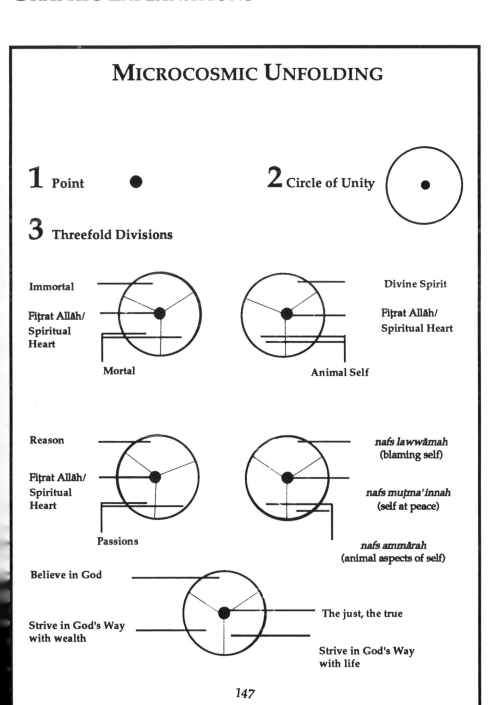

MICROCOSMIC UNFOLDING

1 Point ●

2 Circle of Unity

3 Threefold Divisions

Immortal

Fiṭrat Allāh/
Spiritual
Heart

Mortal

Divine Spirit

Fiṭrat Allāh/
Spiritual Heart

Animal Self

Reason

Fiṭrat Allāh/
Spiritual
Heart

Passions

nafs lawwāmah
(blaming self)

nafs muṭma'innah
(self at peace)

nafs ammārah
(animal aspects of self)

Believe in God

Strive in God's Way
with wealth

The just, the true

Strive in God's Way
with life

147

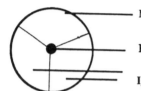

Moral Reasonableness of a Religiously Cultured Monotheist
(*hilm*)

Fiṭrat Allāh/Spiritual Heart

Ignorance (*jahl*)

PERFECTION OF EACH PART PROVIDED BY NATURE

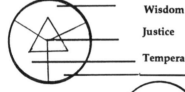

Wisdom

Justice

Temperance   Courage

Balanced,
Centered,
Just,
Spiritual Heart unvelied,
Self at Peace

Movement of Change
Line: Spirit moves in
ascending, descending
and horizontal
motions.

COGNITIVE IMBALANCES: IGNORANCE (*jahl*) OF REALITY

9o

8

1

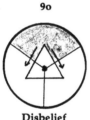 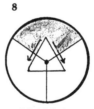 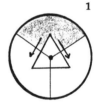

Disbelief
(*kufr*)

Multitheism
(*shirk*)

Hypocrisy
(*nifāq*)

**COGNITIVE BALANCES: MORAL REASONABLENESS OF A RELIGIOUSLY
CULTURED MONOTHEIST (*ḥilm*)**

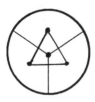 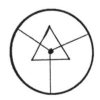

Wisdom
Temperance
Courage

Piety
(*taqwā*)

Justice

SATURN-JUPITER COORDINATIONS

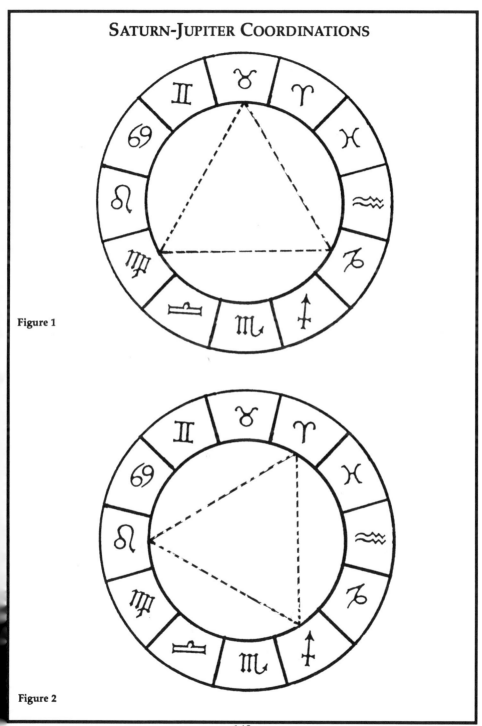

Figure 1

Figure 2

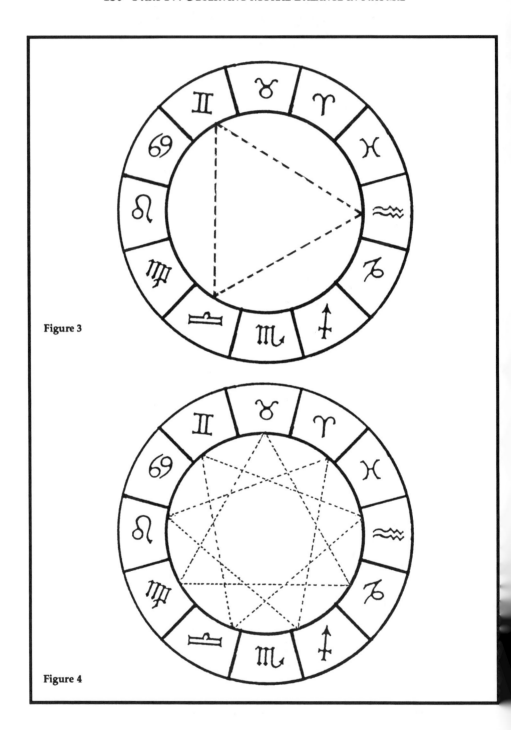

Figure 3

Figure 4

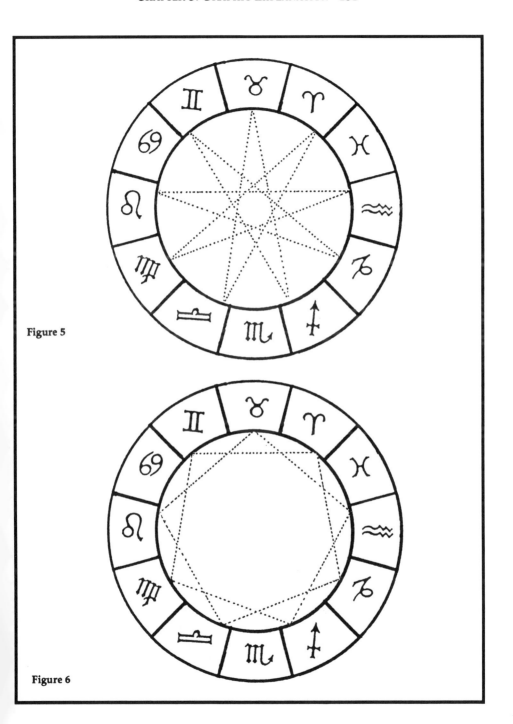

Figure 5

Figure 6

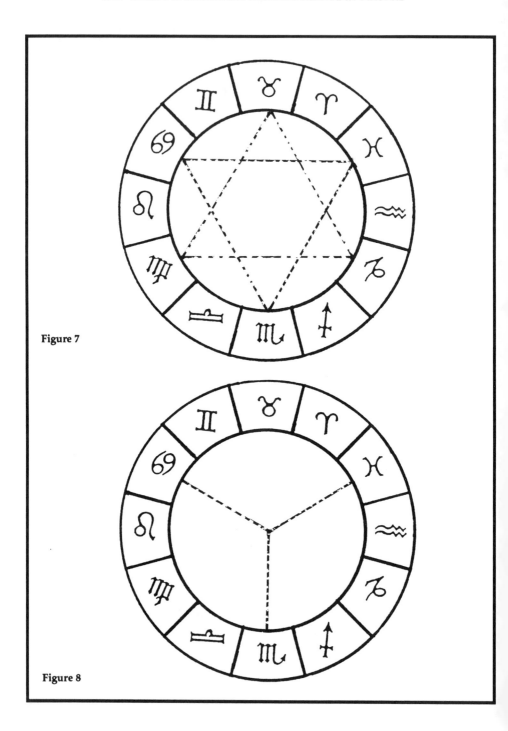

Figure 7

Figure 8

THE ELEMENTAL QUALITIES OF THE ZODIAC

ZODIACAL SIGN	HOT	COLD	WET	DRY
ARIES	X			X
TAURUS		X		X
GEMINI	X		X	
CANCER		X	X	
LEO	X			X
VIRGO		X		X
LIBRA	X		X	
SCORPIO		X	X	
SAGITTARIUS	X			X
CAPRICORN		X		X
AQUARIUS	X		X	
PISCES		X	X	

MICROCOSM-MACROCOSM UNFOLDING

1

•   •

Point

2

Circle of Unity

3

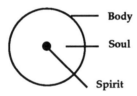

Hidden   Manifest

4

Elements/Qualities   Elements/Qualities

7

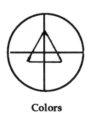

Colors   Colors

12

Throne

Kabah

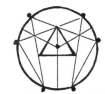

Heart of the Believer

Seven Circumambulations

"...His Throne was upon the Waters" (11:7)

Seven Year Cycles of Saturn and Jupiter

12 into 9

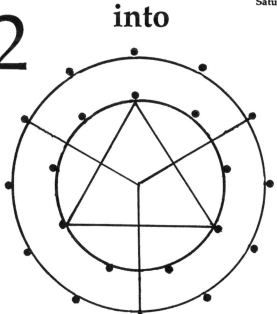

THE TWELVE SIGNS OF THE ZODIAC AND THEIR ELEMENTAL QUALITIES

COLD/WET/DRY

Tarus

Cancer   Pisces

Virgo   Capricorn

Scorpio

HOT/WET/DRY

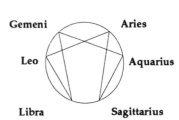

Gemeni   Aries

Leo   Aquarius

Libra   Sagittarius

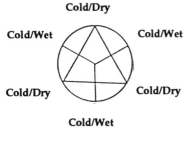

Cold/Dry

Cold/Wet   Cold/Wet

Cold/Dry   Cold/Dry

Cold/Wet

Hot/Wet   Hot/Dry

Hot/Dry   Hot/Wet

Hot/Wet   Hot/Dry

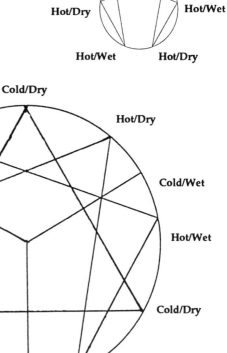

Cold/Dry

Hot/Wet   Hot/Dry

Cold/Wet   Cold/Wet

Hot/Dry   Hot/Wet

Cold/Dry   Cold/Dry

Hot/Wet   Hot/Dry

Cold/Wet

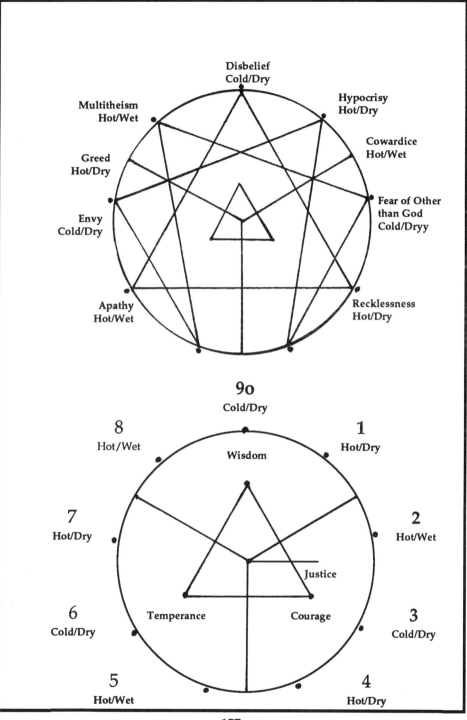

Disbelief
Cold/Dry

Hypocrisy
Hot/Dry

Cowardice
Hot/Wet

Multitheism
Hot/Wet

Greed
Hot/Dry

Fear of Other
than God
Cold/Dryy

Envy
Cold/Dry

Apathy
Hot/Wet

Recklessness
Hot/Dry

90
Cold/Dry

8
Hot/Wet

1
Hot/Dry

Wisdom

7
Hot/Dry

2
Hot/Wet

Justice

6
Cold/Dry

Temperance

Courage

3
Cold/Dry

5
Hot/Wet

4
Hot/Dry

PART V
ATTAINING MORAL BALANCE
THROUGH NURTURE

CHAPTER 1
INTRODUCTION

In addition to the process of nature's method of operation which has given the tools and instruments to guide the self to perfection, the nurturing process also has natural tools and instruments to guide this process. Tools include practical, cognitive, behavioral, affective or humanistic techniques to prevent the development of negative traits.

The goal of the self according to spiritual chivalry is to perfect nature's method of operation by becoming centered, balanced in justice. When the self is thus motivated, it learns to read the Signs of nature and nurture's guidelines as it moves towards this goal. Preservation of the self's natural inclination to balance begins in the home where parents model how to preserve their natural balance by living a centered life themselves. This process has been described extensively in the books on the science of ethics. Having been born in a state of grace in the traditional perspective with no encumbrance of "original sin," it is within human nature to preserve the centered self by actualizing the potential positive traits of its natural disposition.

Methods of preserving the natural state of moral balance include personal effort, endeavor, struggle and appropriate self-training. According to the traditional perspective, the main function of religion is to guide the human being towards completion of the perfection of nature's mode of operation in the self, that is, becoming conscious of self. If the human being were incapable of changing traits acquired through nurture and the environment, there would have been no need for God to send Prophets and His revelation to them. The Prophet of Islam said, "Make your disposition beautiful." Even in nature,

161

according to psychoethics, wild animals can change and be domesticated; a horse can be trained to carry a saddle. If animals can be changed, all the more can the human being change who has the power of reason. Ibn Miskāwayh points out that change does not mean to uproot traits like inappropriate anger and lust, but to control them in a state of moderation as appropriate anger or lust by making them receptive to receiving the spiritual. He points out, however, that the speed of change differs from individual to individual.

Algazel divides people into four types.

> The first group do not distinguish positive from negative traits. They lack conviction of their conscience because of an unfavorable nurturing process. The reason is not that their attraction to pleasure or affective system (feelings) is strong because they are indifferent to pleasures. The personality of such a person may develop positive traits for a short period of time, but they will not be lasting qualities of the self. The second group are those who are aware of the harm to the self that negative traits and actions bring, but do nothing about them because they take pleasure in them. The centering process is more difficult for them in comparison to the first group. They can succeed, however, through strenuous effort. The third group, because of their nurturing process, have come to believe that negative traits are actually positive so they pursue them wholeheartedly. The centering of such a person is considered to be next to impossible. The fourth group are those who in addition to nurturing negative traits and actions, see their own excellence and perfection in them. They are the type who challenge their friends to do something more negative than they have done. They are the most difficult type to achieve centering.[1]

Algazel refers to a saying in regard to this type to the effect: "It is real torture to train a full-grown wolf to be well-mannered."[2]

CHAPTER 2
COGNITIVE TECHNIQUES

GAINING KNOWLEDGE

In order to center the self, cognitive remedies are recommended like gaining knowledge which is also considered to be a religious obligation. Wisdom, one of the four positive dispositions, refers to a person's faith in Reality. This differs from conjecture[1] and mere fancy.[2] Signs pointing to Reality are detailed[3] and explained[4] so that the human being might reflect and think about the different phenomena of nature.[5] Nurture's guidance repeatedly advises the human being to observe the phenomena of nature to arrive at Reality.[6] Ibn Miskāwayh expands on this:

An obligation incumbent on those who seek to preserve a balanced, centered self (moral goodness) is to apply themselves to gaining theoretical as well as practical knowledge—a duty which they should not, under any circumstances, be allowed to neglect so that it may serve the self just as physical exercise is pursued to preserve the health of the body. Physicians ascribe great importance to exercise in the preservation of the health of the body. Physicians of the 'self' attribute even greater importance to it in the preservation of a healthy self. For when the self ceases to speculate and loses the power of thought and of deep searching for meanings, it becomes dull, stupid and devoid of the substance of all positive traits. If it becomes accustomed to laziness, shuns reflection and chooses to remain idle, it draws near to destruction, because, by this idleness, it casts off its particular form and returns to the rank of beasts. This, indeed, is the relapse of character. May God protect us against it!

163

Further, should those who are seeking to preserve this healthy, centered self become unique and eminent in knowledge, then let not their pride in what they have achieved cause them to cease to seek beyond, for knowledge has no limit, and above every human being of knowledge there is One who knows. Let them not be too lazy to review what they have learned and perfected by studying it further, for forgetfulness is the bane of learning. Let them remember the words of al-Hasan al-Basri (may God grant him mercy!) 'Curb your self, for it is inquisitive, and polish it for it quickly becomes rusty.' And let it be known to you that these words, though short, are full of meaning and, at the same time, they are eloquent.[7]

STUDYING MATHEMATICAL SCIENCES

In order to attain this second method, children are instructed to study the mathematical sciences. Ibn Miskāwayh says:

> If youths who are growing up accustom themselves, from the start of their life, to intellectual exercise and pursue the four mathematical sciences, (arithmetic, geometry, music and astronomy), they will become accustomed to truthfulness and will be able to bear the burdens of reflection and speculation. They will delight in the truth. Their character will shun falsehood. Their ears will abhor lying. When they reach their prime and proceed to study philosophy, they will retain the same disposition as they go through it and will absorb from it what should be kept in store. Nothing in philosophy will seem strange to them nor will they need to toil hard to understand its secrets or extract its hidden treasures...[8]

SEEKING WITHIN, NOT WITHOUT

A third method is to seek the divine blessings within rather than material goods.

Again, let those who are seeking to preserve a healthy self

realize that, by so doing, they are indeed preserving noble blessings. These are bestowed upon them like great treasures hidden within them or like splendid garments which are put on them. Let them realize also that if one who possesses such sublime blessings within their 'self' are not obliged to seek these blessings from outside, nor to pay money to others for their sake, nor to endure hardship and burdensome troubles in their pursuit—if they then shun and neglect them to the point of overlooking them, they, indeed, will deserve blame for their actions and will show poor judgment. They will prove to be neither wise nor successful. [Moral-seekers should realize this fact] as they observe how the pursuers of external goods venture on far and perilous journeys, travel frightful and rugged roads, and expose themselves to all kinds of dangers and possibilities of destruction by beasts of prey and wicked aggressors in order to attain material goods. In most cases, even after undergoing all these horrors, such people fail. They may suffer excessive repentance and great sorrow which stifles their breath and severs the members of their body. And even if they attain one of their desires, it may be lost quickly or be exposed to loss. It holds no hope of permanence, since it is external. What is external to us cannot be secure against the innumerable accidents which affect it. At the same time, its owner is in a state of intense fear, constant anxiety, and weariness of body and of the self, trying to keep what can in no way be kept and to watch over something where watchfulness is of no avail.[9]

COUNTING YOUR BLESSINGS

Healthy persons are encouraged to count their blessings.

As for those blessings which are in ourselves, they exist with us and in us. They do not leave us, because they are the gift of God the Creator (mighty and exalted is He!) He has commanded us to put them to use and to

rise higher in their scale. If we follow His commandment, these blessings will yield us [other] blessings in
succession and we will rise from one grade to another
until they lead us to eternal bliss. Who is it, then, who
suffers a worse deal or a more obvious fall than they
who lose precious and lasting gems which are with them
and at their disposal and seek base and perishable
unessentials which are neither with them nor at their
disposal? Even if they happen to obtain the material
things, these things will not remain in their possession to
be left with them, for it is inevitable that either they will
be separated from their things or their things from them.
This is why we have said that those who have been sufficiently provided for and who have gained a moderate
share of external happiness should not be engaged in the
superfluities of life because they are endless and lead
their seekers to endless perils. The true purpose sought
through moderation is the treatment of one's pains and
the avoidance of falling victim to them and not enjoyment and the pursuit of pleasure. For when one treats
hunger and thirst—both of which are incidental diseases
and pains—one should not seek the body's pleasure but,
rather, he should seek its health, and one will get the
pleasure eventually. But one who, through treatment,
seeks pleasure and not health, will neither obtain health
nor keep such pleasure.[10]

BEING SELF-REFLECTIVE

A person should become self-reflective as a method of
preserving a healthy self according to the traditional
view:

> Furthermore, those who wish to preserve the cen-
> tered self should pay minute attention to all of their acts
> and plans in the execution of which they use the organs
> of their body and self, lest they use them by force of pre-
> vious habit which diverges from their judgment and

reflection. How often it happens that people set out to do something which varies from their previous resolution and decision! Whoever finds themselves in this position should fix for themselves penalties to counteract such misdeeds. If for instance they suspect themselves of seeking some kind of harmful food, or failing to adhere to a self-imposed diet, or eating unwholesome fruits or pastries, they should penalize themselves by fasting and should only break their fast by taking the lightest and the smallest amount of food. If they are able to suffer hunger, let them do so and be more strict in their diet even though they may not need such strictness. In reproaching themselves, they may address it as follows: 'You intended to take what is useful to you but you took, instead, what is harmful. Such is the conduct of whoever is devoid of reason. One would think that many animals are better than you because none of them seeks what is pleasurable and then takes what is painful. Hold now yourself, therefore, ready for the penalty.[11]

TRADITIONAL/MODERN TECHNIQUES

Modern psychology has developed numerous cognitive techniques which work with the psychoethical model and examples from the psychology of people like Algazel and Tusī to which reference has already been made. The cognitive system is known to operate through various processes and self-talk is one of them. This is a process which is repeatedly mentioned in psychoethics as the work of the *nafs al-lawwāmah*, the reproaching or blaming aspect of self, which is a function of cognition in centering the self.

Six thoughts and impressions are recommended to be noted down by the moral-seeker. They are: (1) thoughts of physical needs; (2) thoughts of persons considered to be enemies; (3) thoughts of the spirit; (4) thoughts of angels;

(5) thoughts of the cognitive system including reason, free-will and conscience; and (6) intuitive, directly experienced thoughts.[12]

In the view of Jalāl al-Din Rumī, once the moral-seeker consciously expresses the intention to move towards centering or takes action to move towards the positive dispositions of the self, every thought that occurs to him or her is a message from Divine Assistance calling for deep deliberation and a dutiful response. It directs the self to self-knowledge and self-knowledge leads to knowledge of God according to the famous Tradition, "He who knows himself, knows his Lord."[13]

CHAPTER 3
BEHAVIORAL TECHNIQUES

SELF-TRAINING

Algazel describes self-training as struggling with the self until the self's attitudes and behaviors are all in accord with the positive disposition out of habit. This method of change requires perseverance in all voluntary acts of the self which, in turn, include developing will-power and consciousness. The goal is to obtain pleasure in one's positive disposition. Such a person will only be said to have acquired the trait of generosity if he finds joy in giving away his wealth. Constant perseverance is required. Thus an element of will and full consciousness is involved in developing positive traits. According to Algazel, this is the most effective method of making change.

OBSERVATION AND ASSOCIATION

If people associate with others who have positive traits, they will little by little begin to imitate them and develop in a positive way. The most effective learning system for the development of positive traits is through observation and association according to Algazel. As children are more imitative than adults, they pick up the behavior of others very readily and learn in this way. Algazel, Tūsī, Ibn Miskāwayh, Dawwanī have all mentioned the importance of friendships and associations one has with other people.

The importance of friendship as a method of preserving the healthy self has been stressed in nurture's guidance. Humanity was created from a single pair of a male and a female[1] and from a single Divine breath.[2] All believers are brothers[3] and have great love and affection among themselves.[4] Nothing should be allowed to come in the way of doing good or making peace between different persons.[5] Efforts should be made to bring about harmony between people[6] in positive dispositions, not in negative ones.[7] Ibn Miskāwayh explains further:

> When the self has positive traits, loving the acquisition of them and desirous of attaining them, longing for true sciences and for sound knowledge, then its possessor is obligated to associate with those who are akin to themselves and seek those who resemble them, and should not enjoy the presence of others or sit in their company. They should be very careful lest they associate with those defective in morals among the frivolous or among those who display enjoyment of disgraceful pleasures and commitment of inappropriate deeds and boast of them and indulge in them.[8]

The advice is not to fall into the state that the modern Western world promotes. Based on the Quran and *sunnah*, Ibn Miskāwayh says,

> The love of physical pleasures and of bodily relations is inborn in the human being because of his passions (which make the human being imperfect in comparison to angels). We are inclined to them. We covet them by our primitive nature and our original disposition. It is only by means of reason's restraint that we keep ourselves from them, stopping at the limits which reason prescribes to us and contenting ourselves with what is necessary.[9]

When one has found friends who also strive for positive traits (to be elaborated and explained below), the association needs to be based on the natural laws underlying friendship. Ibn Ibn Miskāwayh says:

This involves necessarily pleasant fun, agreeable conversation, the delightful exchange of jokes and the pursuit of pleasures permitted by the Divine Law and determined by reason without going beyond these pleasures to excessive indulgence, or, on the other hand, scorning them and abstaining from them. For to be carried to one of the extremes would be called—if extreme is excess—frivolity, depravity, dissoluteness, and other blameworthy qualities. If the extreme is deficiency, it would be stupidity, sterness, peevishness and similar qualities which are also blameworthy. The mean between these two extremes is the graceful person who is distinguished by cheerfulness, pleasant disposition, and good companionship. However, it is as difficult to achieve the mean in this case as it is with the other positive traits.[10]

MODELING

Modeling is another area emphasized in psychoethics. Here the models are all people who were ethically sound like the Prophets of the Old and New Testaments and the Quran. Modeling is such an important concept in the Quran that people are told to follow the example of God's Messenger. Following his example forms the second most important source for the Divine Law after revelation. This is called the *sunnah* or implementing the actions, customs, and sayings of Muhammad. There is a famous Tradition from him, as well, in regard to four women who are among the most beloved of God. They include Asiyah, the Pharaoh of Egypt's wife who nurtured Moses and turned away from her husband who was a tyrant; the Virgin Mary who gave birth to Jesus; Khadijah, the Messenger's first wife who had been a wealthy widow fifteen years his senior and who spent all of her wealth for the spread of the faith; and Fatimah, the Messenger's youngest daughter who accepted a life rich in the spirit at the same time as it was poor in terms of material comforts.

Ibn Miskāwayh adds:

Furthermore, they who are anxious to preserve a healthy self should follow the example of those leaders who are known for their prudence and foresight in defense against external enemies. It is on this basis that we should establish our means in preparing for such enemies as greed, anger, and all that removes us from the positive traits which we pursue. This preparation consists in accustoming ourselves to being patient where patience is necessary, to forgiving those whom we should forgive, to abstaining from negative desires, and to mastering these negative traits before they rage, for then the task would be very difficult if not utterly impossible.[11]

Psychodynamic theory in the area of psychological imbalances separate from biological illnesses tends to emphasize those aspects of the self that have to do with defense mechanisms (cognitive in the system of psychoethics). In terms of psychoethics, it would be a person in the undevelopment of the cognitive system. A person who is cognitively unconscious of the Presence of God in a state of disbelief, according to spiritual chivalry, is ruled by the self's irrational behavior (the passions) rather than regulating them.

In psychoethics, transference is explained by the idea of a mirror and modeling, associations, and friendships. Although mirroring is discussed in modern psychotherapy as a technique, in psychoethics it is the idea of transference. It is based on a famous Tradition which says, "The person of faith is the mirror of persons of faith."[12]

Free association is another area of commonalty. It is a technique developed by Freud where the client relates not only their symptoms to the analyst, but any and everything that comes into their awareness without trying to make any kind of logical connection. A variation of this is found in traditional medicine as a method of diagnosis where the physician acts through cognition to understand the cause for a physical/psychic illness.

Keeping Anger in a State of Moderation

A further behavioral technique is controlling anger.

Likewise, if they who wish to preserve the healthy self suspect themselves of being aroused to an anger for which there is no reason, or which is directed against an innocent person, or which exceeds what is proper for themselves, then let them react by exposing themselves to a person who is insolent and whom they know to be obscene. Let them suffer to endure that person's abuse; or let them humble himself before someone whom they know to be good but towards whom they had not acted humbly before; or let them impose upon themselves a certain amount of money to give away as alms and make this a vow which they should never fail to execute.[13]

CHAPTER 4
AFFECTIVE TECHNIQUES

The moral-seeker is advised from early training to speak to people according to the measure of their understanding in order to help them move towards the centering process. An aphorism that is also emphasized is, "Nature is the best physician and habit is second nature."[1] These are clear corollaries of the humanistic approaches to counseling, namely, unconditional positive regard, genuineness, and empathy.

If a person suspects themselves to be lazy or neglect any of their interests, let them punish themselves by engaging in some hard labor, or a long prayer, or certain good works which entail toil and fatigue. In brief, let them impose upon themselves certain definite prescriptions which they should consider as duties and punishments that admit of no infringement or compromise, whenever they suspect themselves of violating their reason or transgressing its command. Let them be wary at all times of involving themselves in any negative trait, or of helping a friend in it, or of violating what is right. Let them not consider as slight any of the small faults which they commit, nor try to excuse themselves for them, because this would lead them to serious ones. Whoever is accustomed in his childhood and youth to controlling themselves instead of surrendering to their passions, to being magnanimous when their anger is aroused, to checking their tongue, and to enduring their companions will bear lightly what others, who have not gone through this training, find burdensome.[2]

CHAPTER 5
MIXED TECHNIQUES

BEHAVIORAL/COGNITIVE TECHNIQUES

Studying of the lives of people who had positive traits is a behavioral/cognitive method in addition to observation and association. It is effective when observation and association are not possible.

AFFECTIVE AND BEHAVIORAL TECHNIQUES

Yet another area mentioned to preserve the health of the self is to refrain from stimulating the behavioral and affective aspects of self until they themselves make a demand.

Another requirement which should be observed by whoever is anxious to preserve the healthy self is to refrain from stirring their affective/emotive and behavioral functions by reminding themselves of what they obtained from them and of the pleasure which they have thus experienced through them. They should rather leave them alone until they are stirred by themselves. I mean by this that they may remember the pleasures they had from the satisfaction of their passions and their delightfulness or the grades they have achieved of the honor and glory of authority, and may consequently desire these things. But once they desire them, they move towards them. When they do so they come to regard them as ends. Thus they find themselves drawn to use their power of reflection and to employ their cognitive function to help them attain those ends. This is like the one who arouses beasts of prey and excites wild, rapacious animals and then seeks to appease them and to be delivered from them. Intelligent people do not choose to be in such a situation. This is rather the conduct of fools who do not distinguish between good and evil or between right and wrong. This is why they who are anxious to preserve the healthy self should not remind themselves of the actions of these affective and behavioral functions lest they desire them and seek them. Let them, instead, leave them alone, for they will roused by themselves. They will be excited when necessary and they will seek what the body needs. They will find in the stimulus of nature what will save them the trouble of stimulating these two functions by their thought, reflection and discernment. Their thought and discernment will then be used in satisfying their need and in assessing the freedom that they should give them to ensure what is necessary and requisite for their body to preserve their health. This is the way to execute the will of God (exalted is He!) and to carry out His plan, for He (exalted and sanctified is He!) has endowed us with these two functions, only in order that we use them when we need them and not to become their servants and slaves. Thus, those who put the cognitive function in the service of their own slaves violates God's commandment, transgresses the limits which He has set and reverses His guidance and design. For our Creator (mighty and exalted is He!) has provided us with these functions by His plan and design and no justice could be nobler or superior to that of His provision and design. Anyone who opposes it [His justice] or deviates from it commits the greatest wrong and injustice towards his own self.[1]

PART VI
ATTAINING MORAL BALANCE THROUGH THE SIGN OF THE PRESENCE OF GOD

CHAPTER 1
THE HEALING WORK

CHANGE

No matter how positive one's nurturing process has been, negative traits will have slipped in to cloud over the mirror of the spiritual aspects of the heart. These negative traits form what is called the false self. However, just as nature provides means through nurture to limit the development of the false self, it also provides the means to morally heal. This change, in the traditional view, is possible to achieve through greater struggle (*jihād al-akbar*) and divine grace or assistance. As we never know when Divine Grace may come, once conscious of negative traits, we then begin the struggle to overcome the false self.

Algazel suggests three methods the awakened one can pursue. First, ask a truthful friend who is pious and who has insight to point out one's negative traits. Such a friend is hard to find. Most people prefer not to point out the negative traits of a friend because that leaves them open for the awareness of their own negative traits. Second, if one not have an honest friend, ask one's enemy who will readily state one's negative traits. Third, mix with people who are not afraid to ascribe to themselves the negative traits that they see in the other person. Algazel says that whenever a person perceives any negative trait in another, he should suspect its presence in himself to a greater or lesser degree and begin to reflect on himself.

LEVELS OF
RESTORATION TO MORAL BALANCE

General rules of restoration to moral balance are mentioned by Tusī who then mentions four specific techniques.

> The systems of the self are confined to three areas, as we have said: the cognitive system, the attraction to pleasure and the avoidance of harm. Since, again, the imbalances of each occur in two kinds, either through a imbalance in the quantity of the system or through an imbalance in its quality; and since, moreover, the imbalance in quantity represents either a departure from equilibrium in the direction of overdevelopment or a departure from equilibrium in the direction of underdevelopment, therefore, the imbalances of each system may be of three sorts in conformity with overdevelopment, with underdevelopment, or with undevelopment.
>
> These are the classes of simple moral imbalances occurring in the systems of the self, of which there are many species; and many other moral imbalances arise from compounds thereof, all of which derive, however, from these classes. Among these imbalances there are some which are called 'fatal' and most of the chronic imbalances have their origins therein: these cover such cases as overconsciousness of self leading to perplexity and ignorance in the theoretical intellect, while in the case of the other systems such things are involved as anger, cowardice, fear of other than God, sadness, envy, desire, passion and sloth. The harm these disorders inflict on the self is all the more serious, and their method of restoration to balance (accordingly) more important and more generally beneficial. [1]

In addition to general methods of restoration to balance, four specific stages are also given, depending upon the extent of the imbalance. These four categories or stages are exactly the same four used by traditional physicians in treating physical illnesses.

> General remedies in medicine are effected by the use of

four categories of treatment: diet, medication, poison, and cauterization or surgery. In psychical disorders, too, one must make use of the same system.[2]

The first stage of treatment to be used if the imbalance is at a relatively early stage of development is diet. A general description of this stage of restoration to moral balance, beginning with consciousness and awareness of the human imperfection, is given by Tūsī.

> One should first clearly recognize the harm of the negative trait one seeks to change [i.e., gain cognitive consciousness of it]. There should be no doubt about it in order to have the necessary motivation to effect change. One should become aware though imagery of the harmful effects the negative trait has on the self whether in one's faith or in one's worldly affairs. Then, at the next stage one should shun the learned negative trait by the use of will-power. If one's purpose is attained, well and good. If not, one must constantly concern oneself with the application of the positive trait corresponding to that negative one, going to great lengths to repeat, in the most excellent way and the fairest manner, the acts pertaining to that function. Such remedies, generally speaking, correspond to treatment by diet as practiced by physicians.[3]

The second stage in medical practice is the use of medication. An equivalent method is employed in traditional psychotherapy in dealing with the unconsciously learned negative traits of the preconscious, unconscious self. Tūsī explains:

> If, however, by this sort of imbalance [i.e., diet] the imbalance is not balanced, one must proceed to consciously chide and revile, to humiliate and reproach the self for the act in question, either in thought or by word or deed. If this does not produce the desired result [of

the negative trait changing to centering and use of the positive trait] and one's purpose is to adjust one of either the two functions—behavioral [anger to ward off pain and survive] or affective/emotive [lust to preserve the human species], then one must effect this change by the use of the other function, for whenever one is dominate, the other is dominated. Moreover, just as the natural, created purpose of the affective/emotive function is to preserve alive the individual and the species, so the purpose of the behavioral function is to defeat the onslaught of "attraction to pleasure."Thus, when they neutralize and compensate each other, the cognitive function has scope for distinction. This category of restoration to balance is analogous to the giving of medication by medical physicians.[4]

The third category or stage of restoration to moral balance, that of poison, is used medically to effect change when the negative habit is firmly entrenched and deep-rooted in the self.

If, again, the imbalance is not eliminated by this method [i.e., medication], ... then, in order to crush it, one must seek help from the entrenched negative trait by consciously developing the opposite negative trait. However, one must always closely observe the condition of the self and notice any adjustment made in the condition. That is to say, when the [deeply entrenched] negative trait begins to decline [in terms of intensity] and approaches the mean, which is the place of the positive trait, the moral-seeker must abandon the course on which he has embarked in order not to incline from equilibrium to the other end of the continuum and thereby fall into another imbalance. This category of restoration to moral balance corresponds to the poisonous remedy to which the medical physician does not put his hand unless he is compelled to do so; and when he does, he recognizes the obligation to careful observa-

tion and monitoring the disorder so that there be no
declination of the one disorder towards its opposite.
'As for him who fears to stand in the presence of his
Lord and keeps the self from passion, then surely paradise—that is his abode.' Prophetic traditions too command resisting the passions. The teaching of the Divine
Law also. The Divine Law also enjoined the removal of
negative traits from the self by good acts of the body.
This constitutes the source of the specific form of opposition found in the ethics of Ghazali, etc., that is, the
removal of a negative trait by removing its causes and
the removal of causes by means of their opposites.[5]

Makki says:

Know that the negative traits of the self are their
imbalances and the moral healing of the self is through
a remedy... For every moral imbalance of the self there
is a remedy commensurate with the smallness or greatness of the imbalance. Apply, then, a remedy for the
imbalance wherever it attacks you, by introducing the
antidote of the disease or by cutting off its root.[6]

The fourth stage of restoration to moral balance is
known as cauterization or surgery and just as this is the
last stage of treatment of medical diseases, so too with
moral imbalance.

If this type of restoration to moral balance [i.e., poi-
son], too, proves insufficient, the self constantly returning to the repetition of the [same deep-rooted] negative
trait, then it must be consciously chastised and dead-
ened. Difficult and arduous tasks must be imposed
upon it to effect change. Furthermore, one should set
about making vows and covenants that are difficult to
implement after becoming aware of the negative effects
upon the self. This category of restoration to moral balance is like the cutting-off of limbs in medicine or the

cauterization of the extremities. The final remedy is
surgery. [7]

The following imbalances are described as imbalances
in quantity producing an over or underdevelopment of a
positive disposition or an imbalance in quality which produces an undevelopment (o) of a positive disposition.

> The goal of self in psychoethics is unity (*tawhid*)
> which is achieved by the self when it completes the per-
> fection of nature in its mode of operation in the self. As
> the self seeks balance, it learns to read the Signs of
> *takwīnī* [guidance through creation] and *tashr'ī* [guid-
> ance through nature] on the way to completing the per-
> fection of nature in its mode of operation. The stages are:
> becoming conscious of self; becoming centered in posi-
> tive traits; benefiting another person; and practicing
> guiding the development of positive traits and prevent-
> ing the development of negative ones in other and in the
> self.[8]

Tūsī explains:

> It must be understood that the professional rule in
> treating imbalances is as follows, first, to know the class-
> es of imbalances, then to recognize their causes and
> symptoms, and finally to proceed to restoration thereof.
> Moreover, imbalances are constitutional declinations
> from (a state of) equilibrium, while their treatment is the
> restoration of such constitutions to equilibrium by tech-
> nical skill.[9]

Each one of the three segments of the self–cognition
(C), avoidance of harm/pain (B), and attraction to pleasure (A) have a positive trait. The positive traits—courage,
wisdom and temperance—could have three possible states
of imbalances or negative traits. The tendency towards the
development and perfection of the positive traits is consid-

ered the goal of the human being's natural disposition whereas negative traits are considered to be imperfections and a result of an imbalance attained from the nurturing process.

Now since the systems of the self are confined to three areas, as we have said: the cognitive system, the attraction to pleasure and the avoidance of harm. Since, again, the imbalances of each occur in two kinds, either through an imbalance in the quantity of the system or through an imbalance in its quality; and since, moreover, the disorder in quantity represents either a departure from equilibrium in the direction of overdevelopment or in a departure from equilibrium in the direction of underdevelopment, therefore, the imbalances of each system may be of three sorts in conformity with overdevelopment, with underdevelopment, or with undevelopment.[10]

THE SIGN OF THE PRESENCE OF GOD

The Sign, as we have seen, is a circle divided into nine equal parts with a number—1, 2, 4, 5, 7, and 8 placed on the circumference, the farthest distance from the center, representing imbalances in terms of quantity. Three numbers, namely, 3o, 6o, and 9o, are on the outside edge of the circumference indicating an even further distance from the center. They indicate an imbalance in terms of quality. Around the center point is a triangle containing three numbers, namely, 3*, 6* and 9* representing balance. The circle is divided clockwise starting on the right into three segments: avoidance of harm/pain/behavior (B), attraction to pleasure/affect (A), and cognition (C) at the top. 3* stands for the perfection of avoidance of harm/pain or courage (trust in God). 6* stands for the perfection of the attraction to pleasure/affect or temperance (charity towards others). 9* stands for the perfection of cognition or wisdom (belief in the One God). The final aspect of the design to be noted is what is referred to as the movement of change line which moves 1 to (3*) to 4 to (3*) to 2 to (9*) to 8 to (6*) to 5 to (6*) to 7 to (9*) and back to 1. This movement of change line tells how to treat each moral imbalance at four different levels. It is arrived at by dividing 1 by 7, 2 by 7, 3 by 7, 4 by 7, 5 by 7, and 6 by 7.

The first level (diet) is for the imbalance to be moved towards the positive trait in the neighboring segment: attraction to pleasure (A), avoidance of harm/pain (B) or cognition (C). The second level (medication) is to move to the second positive trait on the way to the third number and its segment. The third level (poison) is to move to the number at the end of the line and the negative trait it represents. Here the negative trait is used as treatment because this is the stage of 'poison'. Surgery is to move the entire segment towards the positive trait in a neighboring segment. With cognitive imbalances, level 1 (diet) and level 2 (medication) are treated with the same positive trait. The imbalance in quality (3o, 6o, or 9o) have only two stages of treatment because they are so firmly entrenched in the self: poison or surgery.

CHAPTER 2: COGNITIVE IMBALANCES

(8)
UNDERDEVELOPMENT OF WISDOM

Traits of cognitive imbalance (8) result in the following states of being:

Ignorant
Mistrustful
Multitheist
Preconscious of Reality
Prejudiced
Satanic Temptations, Influenced by

Levels of Restoration to Moral Balance

The negative trait of preconsciousness of Reality can be recognized by the fact that it is a state of the self which prevents the avoidance of harm/pain or attraction to pleasure reaching the necessary amount to preserve the individual or the species. It is to not know and know that one does not know.

Moving towards temperance at levels 1 (diet) and 2 (medication) you need to study nature closely and see how animals are capable of the amount of perception needed to deal with their daily life and preserve the species. Lacking the ability to do this when one has the potential is to disregard an important aspect of humanness.

Level 1 (Diet)/Level 2 (Medication): To move from underdevelopment of cognition (8) towards the center of the attraction to pleasure system or temperance (6*) which is described as being marked by moderation—not being extreme or excessive in either attachment to this world or lack of attachment.

Level 3 (Poison): To move from underdevelopment of cognition (8) to underdevelopment of avoidance of harm/pain (2) which is characterized by being cowardly. Entering this stage of restoration to moral balance is very dangerous and must be carefully monitored so that one negative trait not replace another. Once movement is noticed, this treatment should stop.

Level 4 (Surgery): Sublimate energies of the cognitive system to the attraction to pleasure system by getting in touch with pleasures that do not require any thinking. Once movement is noticed, they can continue as they may increase positive energies but they should not be done in excess after the temporary period of "surgery" to the detriment of one's other responsibilities like seeing to the needs of one's family or earning a legitimate livelihood which also foster moral healing.

Movement of Change Line:

Diet/Medication: 1 (C) to 6* (A)

Poison: 1 (C) to 2 (B)

Surgery: 1 (C) to (A)

Example: Preconsciousness of Reality, in the view of spiritual chivalry, results in multitheism, the worship of more gods than there are. It arises out of a state of ignorance of Reality. The multitheist comes to believe that forces other than God have a role in directing the affairs of the world. It is to immerse self in the material world becoming forgetful of Reality. This type of person, in the view of spiritual chivalry, is a believer in the existence of more than One God. This is considered to be in a state of ignorance of Reality. On the outside, it leads to racial, class and gender discrimination while on the inside it is to follow the idol/ego within dividing the self from its nature originated by God. "...*having hearts with which they under-*

stand not and having eyes with which they see not and having ears with which they hear not. These are as the cattle—nay, they are worse. These are the neglectful" (7:179).

(1)

OVERDEVELOPMENT OF WISDOM

The dictionary includes the following states of being:

Conjecture
Contemptuous
Crafty
Cunning
Deceitful
Doubtful
Excessive Speech
False Promises, Make (see Deceit)
Foolish
Hypocrite
Liar
Malicious
Ostentatious (see Showing Off)
Overconscious of Human Self
Perplexed
Showing Off
Shrewd (see Cunning)
Slanderer
Sly (see Cunning)
Wily (see Cunning)

Levels of Restoration to Moral Balance

Level 1/2 (Diet/Medication): To move from overdevelopment of cognition (1) towards the center of the avoidance of harm/pain or courage (3*) which is described as mental or moral strength to venture, persevere and withstand danger, fear or difficulty.

Level 3 (Poison): To move from overdevelopment of cognition (1) to overdevelopment of attraction o pleasure (7) characterized by love of the world. Entering this stage is very dangerous and should be carefully monitored so that one negative trait not replace another. Once movement is noticed, this treatment should stop.

Level 4 (Surgery): Sublimate energies of the overdevelopment of the cognitive system to the attraction to pleasure system by getting in touch with pleasures that do not require any thinking. Once movement is noticed, you can continue as you may increase positive energies but you should not do so in excess after the temporary period of "surgery" to the detriment of your other responsibilities like seeing to the needs of your family or earning a legitimate livelihood which also fosters moral healing.

Movement of Change Line:
Diet/Medication: 1 (C) to 3* (B)
Poison: 1 (C) to 7 (A)
Surgery: 1 (C) to (A)

Explanation: Allowing the avoidance of harm/pain and attraction to pleasure systems to together rule the self because of the weakness of one's reasoning powers, this type of imbalance for the spiritual warrior is that of being a hypocrite. In defining hypocrisy, there are two basic types: behavioral and verbal. Behavioral hypocrisy is to give an impression of friendship and affection and pretend to be sincere and sympathetic while in one's heart one harbors the opposite feeling. It is to behave one way when the person is present and another when that person is absent. Verbal hypocrisy is to praise and flatter someone whenever one meets them, appearing to be a friend, but denouncing them and speaking slanderously of them in their absence.

In the Quran Satan says to Adam and Eve, *"Lo! I am a sincere advisor to you"* (7:21) while being the opposite of what he claimed. The only objective of a hypocrite is his own personal benefit and the only goal is self-aggrandizement. It is the opposite of truthfulness, sincerity, magnanimity and courage. The hypocrite *"severs that which God has commanded and should be joined and makes mischief in the earth. There is a curse and theirs is the ill abode"* (13:25)

Hypocrisy leads to worse moral traits which are compound imbalances like slandering, backbiting, divulging a believer's secrets, and so forth.

Restoration to Moral Balance: The behavioral technique of systematic desensitization is useful. Imagine the harms that proceed from this negative trait. If people know one is a hypocrite, one will be degraded in the eyes of his or her friends. They will avoid his or her company and he or she will be deprived of his or her friendship. For anyone who has a sense of honor and dignity endowed with a conscience, they need to eliminate this negative trait from self.

The second method is also behavioral and based on self-monitoring. Spiritual warriors need to be vigilant in regard to their acts so that they deliberately act against their desires, waging war against the false self inwardly as well as outwardly in deed and in speech. They need to concentrate on noting their behavior irregardless of affect.

(90)
UNDEVELOPMENT OF WISDOM

The negative traits are the following states of being:

Atheist (see Disbeliever)
Denial
Disbeliever
Fatalist
Identification
Inconstancy in Affairs
Introjection
Isolation
Narcotization

Projection
Rationalization
Reaction Formation
Remission in Important Affairs
Repression
Superstitious (see Unconscious)
Unconscious

Levels of Restoration to Moral Balance

The levels of treatment are twofold: either Level 3 (Poison) or Level 4 (Surgery). Level 3 (Poison) is to move towards underdevelopment (8) or overdevelopment (1) of cognition before any other treatment can be undertaken and then follow the healing methods of the cognitive system (preconsciousness or overconsciousness) until one is centered in wisdom (belief in the One God).

Level 4 (Surgery) is to move directly to wisdom (9*) described by spiritual chivalry as having a wise attitude or taking a wise course of action as the trustee of nature. This is to move in a great leap from total absence of quality to quality without moving through quantity.

Movement of Change Line:
Poison: 9(o) to 8 (C) or 1 (C)
Surgery: 9(o) to 9* (C)

Explanation: The causes of this moral imbalance have been dealt with elsewhere in this handbook. They are basically ingratitude towards God and covering over the truth of Reality.

CHAPTER 3: AVOIDANCE OF HARM/PAIN IMBALANCES

(2)

UNDERDEVELOPMENT OF COURAGE

The underdevelopment negative traits are the following states of being

Anger, Lack of Necessary (see Cowardly)
Bashful
Conceal the Truth
Cowardly
Deserter
Dignity, Lack of a Sense of
Faint-hearted (see Cowardly)
Humiliation of One's Self and/or Family
Inferiority Complex
Nervous
Self-Abasing
Self-Confidence, Lacking in
Self-Conscious (see Bashful)
Self-Debasing (see Self-Abasing)
Self-Degrading (see Self-Abasing)
Self-Demeaning (see Self-Abasing)
Self-Esteem, Lack of
Self-Humiliating (see Self-Abasing)
Self-Regard, Lack of (see Self-Esteem, Lack of)
Spiritless
Timid (see Bashful)

Levels of Restoration to Moral Balance

Level 1 (Diet): To move from underdevelopment of avoidance of harm/pain (2) towards the center of cognition or wisdom (9*) which is described as having a wise attitude or taking a wise course of action as the trustee of nature. It may be knowledge based, insight based or judgment based in common sense.

Level 2 (Medication): To move from underdevelopment of avoidance of harm/pain (2) towards the center of attraction to pleasure (6*) or temperance which is described as being marked by moderation—not being extreme or excessive in either attachment to the world or lack of attachment.

Level 3 (Poison): To move from underdevelopment of avoidance of harm/pain (2) to its other extreme of overdevelopment (4) which is characterized by excessive or inappropriate anger. Entering this stage of restoration to health is very dangerous and must be carefully monitored so that one negative trait not replace another. Once movement is noticed, this treatment should stop.

Level 4 (Surgery): Sublimate energies from the avoidance of harm/pain system to the cognitive system through increasing remembrance (*dhikr*) and prayer. Once movement is noticed, remembrance and prayer can continue as they increase positive energies but they should not be done in excess after the temporary period of "surgery" to the detriment of one's other responsibilities like seeing to the needs of one's family or earning a legitimate livelihood which also foster moral healing.

Movement of Change Line:

Diet:	2 (B) to 9* (C)
Medication:	2 (B) to 6* (A)
Poison:	2 (B) to 4 (B)
Surgery:	2 (B) to (C)

Explanation: Lack of the sufficient development of the avoidance of harm function or courage. Taking being cowardly as an example of a 2 imbalance, if the moral-seekers recognize having this imbalance, they are probably at the level of requiring a dietary intervention. Say, for instance, they are able to recognize and speak of the fact that when someone shouts at them, they cower and turn inward not being able to respond. It is to show timidity under circumstances that call for violent action or the lack of the tendency in the self to chastise on occasions where such a tendency is desirable. It also results in humiliation and a miserable life in being at the mercy of one's relatives, children and those with whom they have dealings. It shows a lack of steadfastness in situations that require patience. They become subservient to others. It leads to self-abasement whereby the unjust are empowered to practice injustice. It is to become weak charactered people who act according to impressions that their imagination may produce.

Generally weakness is a negative trait in the self. It is wrong to show weakness in face of difficulties or to lose heart;[1] to be weak in will;[2] to be weary and fainthearted;[3] to be afraid of men;[4] or of Satan.[5]

Moral-seekers move from this position of being cowardly towards 9* or the cognitive system and wisdom. Through self-talk, they should awaken themselves to a sense of shamelessness of this situation. Appropriate anger is like a fire which in this case has gone out but its embers are still ready to be ignited by fanning and blowing.

If being cowardly is at Level 2 where they recognize it to be there but cannot speak about it, they need a medicative intervention. They would move towards 6* or temperance feeling a sense of empathy, unconditional self-regard for themselves and the situation in which they find themselves.

The level of restoration to moral balance of poison would be used when they find that no matter how often the situation repeats itself, they are not able to respond.

Using this level of restoration to moral balance, they would move to 4, the overdevelopment of the avoidance of harm/pain system and use behavioral techniques like systematic desensitization or behavioral rehearsal. They would stimulate anger and a violent temper in themselves and take a violent course of action which is not too dangerous until the self attains a sense of courage to respond appropriately when someone shouts at them. They must be on their guard not to move out of the state of moderation once attained.

If this level of treatment does not work, they need to move towards "surgery" which in this case of an underdevelopment of the avoidance of harm/pain system means you would turn towards the cognitive system and increase prayer and remembrance (*dhikr*).

(4)

OVERDEVELOPMENT OF COURAGE

Falling into 4, the negative traits of the overdevelopment of the avoidance of harm/pain are the following states of being:

Anger, Inappropriate
Annoying
Argumentative/Quarrelsomeness
Arrogant
Conceited
Enmity
Fanatic
Hard-hearted
Harsh
Hasty
Hostile
Ill-tempered
Impatient

Irritable
Joker
Language, Foul
Patronizing
Presumptuous
Pride (see the Proud)
Reckless
Revengeful
Selfish
Treacherous
Troublemaker
Unkind
Vain
Vindictive

Levels of Restoration to Moral Balance

Level 1 (Diet): To move from overdevelopment of avoidance of harm/pain (4) towards the center of avoidance of harm/pain or courage (3*) which is described as mental or moral strength to venture, persevere, and withstand danger, fear or difficulty because of one's trust in God.

Level 2 (Medication): To move from overdevelopment of avoidance of harm/pain to the center of cognition or wisdom (9*) which is described as a wise attitude or taking a wise course of action in spiritual chivalry. It may be knowledge based, insight based or judgment based in common sense.

Level 3 (Poison): To move from overdevelopment of avoidance of harm/pain (4) to overdevelopment of cognition (1) which is characterized by overconsciousness. Entering this stage of restoration to moral balance is very dangerous and must be closely monitored so that one negative trait not replace another. Once movement is noticed, this treatment should stop.

Level 4 (Surgery): Sublimate energies from the overdevelopment of the avoidance of harm/pain system to the cognitive system through increasing remembrance (*dhikr*) and prayer. Once movement is noticed, remembrance and prayer can continue as they increase positive energies but they should not be done in excess after the temporary period of "surgery" to the detriment of one's other responsibilities like seeing to the needs of one's family or earning a legitimate livelihood which also foster moral healing.

Movement of Change Line:

Diet:	4 (B) to 3* (B)
Medication:	4 (B) to 9* (C)
Poison:	4 (B) to 1 (C)
Surgery:	4 (B) to (C)

Example: Causes include: Vanity, Boastfulness, Bickering, Importunity, Jesting, Self-conceit, Derision/ Scorn, Perfidy/ Treachery; Wrongfulness; Seeking Fame; Desire; Revenge; Conceit; Contention and Quarrelsomeness; Jesting; Arrogance; Scorn; Treachery; Unfairness; Quest of Precious Things; Rivalry; Envy; Yearning for Vengeance; Pride; Selfishness; Stubbornness.

Say, for instance, you have a problem controlling your inappropriate anger. You are often led to reckless behavior when you are scorned by your friends and your enemies become overjoyed. It reaches the point where you are physically suffering, as well. If you can talk about it, try the diet treatment which is to move towards 3* or courage. Using the behavioral techniques of self-training, try to achieve complete freedom from inappropriate anger. Reduce the strength of your inappropriate anger. Sit down if you are standing up and lie down if sitting because being close to the earth creates a sense of self-abasement by which vanity, a cause of anger, is removed. It also reduces the heat of anger. Put cold water on your face to lessen body heat.

If medication is required, move towards 9* and cognition. Through self-talk, consider how unseemly excessive anger is. Think carefully before embarking on any particular course of action to see whether reason and religion approve of it or not. If it meets their approval, one may act upon it, but one must abstain if it is disapproved by either of them. It may even be necessary for the self to abstain from actions in which the amount of danger is not great so as to curtail his propensity for anger.

If "poison" is required, move towards the overdevelopment of cognition (1) characterized by overconsciousness which leads you to doubt and perplexity. In this way you begin to doubt yourself, lessening your sense of pride or vanity which are among the causes of inappropriate anger.

At the level of "surgery" you need to sublimate your energies to the cognitive system and increase your remembrance (*dhikr*) and prayer.

(30)
UNDEVELOPMENT OF COURAGE

The 30 imbalances are the following states of being:

Anxiety
Delighting in the Misfortune of Others
Fear
Fear of Death
Fear of Other Than God
Injustice, Toleration of

Levels of Restoration to Moral Balance

The levels of treatment for a 30 imbalance are either poison or surgery because undevelopment represents an imbalance in quality which indicates a lack of the positive quality altogether. Neglect and undevelopment of the positive trait of courage has become so great that depravity has set in along with the almost total loss of ability to avoid harm/pain.

Say, for instance, you often find yourself in a state of

fear—an uneasy expectation that something unpleasant might happen. Using "poison," you move either toward overdevelopment (4) of the avoidance of harm/pain or towards underdevelopment (2). 4 is characterized by inappropriate anger and 2 by being cowardly until one is centered in courage.

With surgery, you may move directly from fear to courage through the use of behavioral techniques like systematic desensitization. In a relaxed state, you imagine that which you fear to the point you can cope with it. If it becomes too painful, stop, relax and visualize again.

Both of these levels of treatment are dangerous and should be carefully monitored.

Movement of Change Line:

Poison: 3o (B) to 2 (B) or 4 (B)

Surgery: 3o (B) to (B)

Chapter 4: Attraction to Pleasure Imbalances

(5)

Underdevelopment of Temperance

Negative traits of underdevelopment include the following states of being:

Apathy in Regard to Food, Sex, Earning a Living
Begrudge
Complacent
Despair
Dissimulation
Impassive (see Apathy)
Indifferent (see Apathy)
Languid, too
Lazy
Lust, Lack of Necessary
Miserly
Obstinate
Retreating from Life (see Apathy)
Self-Restraint, Excessive
Slothful (see Lazy)
Sluggishness of Appetite
Stingy
Stolid (see Impassive)
Stubborn
Unemotional (see Impassiveness)
Unsociable

Levels of Restoration to Moral Balance

Level 1 (Diet): To move from underdevelopment of attraction to pleasure (5) towards the center of attraction to pleasure or temperance (6*) which is described as being marked by moderation—not being extreme or excessive.

Level 2 (Medication): To move from underdevelopment of attraction to pleasure (5) to being centered in cognition or wisdom (9*) which is described as having a wise attitude or taking a wise course of action. It may be knowledge based, insight based or judgment based in common sense.

Level 3 (Poison): To move from underdevelopment of attraction to pleasure (5) to underdevelopment of cognition (8) which is characterized by preconsciousness described as knowing that one does not know. Entering this stage of treatment is very dangerous and must be carefully monitored so that one negative trait does not replace another. Once movement is noticed, this treatment should stop.

Level 4 (Surgery): Sublimate energies of the attraction to pleasure system (affect/emotion) to the avoidance of harm/pain (behavior) system through fasting, avoiding sex, shopping and any thing that attracts one to this world. Once movement is noticed, this treatment can continue because they may increase positive energies but they should not be done in excess after the temporary period of "surgery" to the detriment of one's other responsibilities like seeing to one's family's needs or earning a legitimate livelihood which also foster moral healing.

Movement of Change Line:

Diet:	5 (A) to 6* (A)
Medication:	5 (A) to 9* (C)
Poison:	5 (A) to 8 (C)
Surgery:	5 (A) to (B)

Example: For instance, moral-seekers may suffer from the moral negative trait of miserliness. It is a kind of enslavement of the self and is less curable than extravagance or prodigality. It shows an inordinate love of wealth so that a person is strongly attached to worldly things and this, in turn, hinders centering the self and moral healing.

It should be noted, however, that this trait may be positive or negative. If one appears miserly because of poverty, this is a positive trait. If it is because of excessive love of worldly things, it is a negative trait. At Level 1, you should move towards 6* or temperance, exercising self-restraint but not excessively. It is to develop unconditional positive regard for others and desiring to help them. One way is by gaining intellectual influence. Miserliness will disappear and the love of influence will replace it. This then needs to be removed. Know that the purpose of wealth is to meet one's basic needs so excess should be given away. Guard against acquiring wealth in ways that are unlawful, doubtful, or contrary to humanity. Preserve the necessary amount for self and give the excess to the needy. Give them when they approach. Be cautious in spending. Be content with spending little for the self and moderate amounts for others. Have the correct intention in acquisition, preservation and expenditure.

(7)

OVERDEVELOPMENT OF TEMPERANCE

The negative traits are the following states of being:

Avaricious (see Greedy)
Covetous (see Greedy)
Debasement of Aspiration
Earnings, Illegitimate
Extravagant (see Prodigal)
Gluttonous
Greedy
Hoard
Impudent

Licentious (see Lust)
Loss of Self-Respect
Love of the World (see Love of Wealth and Riches)
Love of Wealth and Riches
Lust
Overbearing
Prodigal
Self-Indulgent
Sexually Harass
Shameless
Spendthrift (see Prodigal)
Squanderer (see Extravagant)
Status Seeking
Wasteful (see Prodigal)
Whimsical

Levels of Restoration of Moral Balance

Level 1 (Diet): To move from overdevelopment of attraction to pleasure (7) towards the center of cognition or wisdom (9*) described in spiritual chivalry as having a wise attitude or taking a wise course of action based on belief in the One God. It may be knowledge based, insight based or judgment based in common sense.

Level 2 (Medication): To move from overdevelopment of the attraction to pleasure (7) system toward the center of avoidance of harm/pain (3*) or courage described as mental or moral strength to venture, persevere, and withstand danger, fear or difficulty based on trust in God.

Level 3 (Poison): To move from overdevelopment of attraction to pleasure (7) to the other extreme of underdevelopment (5) which is characterized by miserliness. Entering this stage of treatment is very dangerous and should be carefully monitored so that one negative trait not replace another. Once movement is noticed, this treatment should stop.

Level 4 (Surgery): Sublimate energies of the attraction to pleasure system (affect/emotion) to the avoidance of harm/pain (behavior) system through fasting, avoiding sex, shopping and anything that attracts one to this world. Once movement is noticed, this treatment can continue because it may increase positive energies but it should not be done in excess after the temporary period of "surgery" to the detriment of one's other responsibilities like seeing to one's family's needs or earning a legitimate livelihood which also foster moral healing.

Movement of Change Line:

Diet:	7 (A) to 9* (C)
Medication:	7 (A) to 3* (B)
Poison:	7 (A) to 5 (A)
Surgery:	7 (A) to (B)

Explanation: Inappropriate lust is one of the negative traits of the attraction to pleasure system. It results in loss of respect by others and loss of piety, as well as the development of greed and delving in futile and frivolous matters which are of no use in this world.

At Level 1 (Diet), move towards 9* and cognition. Divert your thoughts from this negative trait by occupying yourself with the exact sciences like mathematics—disciplines associated with reflection. Recognize that things of this world are transitory and what remains for the self are spiritual attainments. Recognize that the similarity of opposite sex partner outside the bounds of marriage is like leaving a deliciously prepared meal uneaten in one's home and begging at the door of other houses in search of that which will relieve the pangs of hunger. Through self-talk, show the self that it is a useless pursuit.

At level 2, move towards the behavioral system and courage. Associate with friends who have discernment. Still the lust by coition or use of depressants. Take a lengthy journey. Burden the self with arduous exercise or enterprises. Embark upon difficult tasks.

At Level 3 (Poison) cultivate miserliness (5) until you sense that you have moved closer to temperance (6*).

At Level 4 (Surgery), abstain from food and drink so

weakness overtakes the physical faculties but without leading to collapse.

(60)

Undevelopment of Temperance

Negative traits include the following states of being:
Backbite
Envious
Grieving
Sad (see Grieving)

Levels of Restoration to Moral Balance

Treatment is either through "poison" (Level 3) or "surgery" (Level 4). At Level 3, it is either to move towards underdevelopment (5) of the attraction to pleasure or overdevelopment (7) and then follow the healing methods of either. At level 4, surgery, you need to move towards temperance (6*)

Movement of the Line of Change:

Poison: 60 (A) to 5 (A) or 7 (A)
Surgery: 60 (A) to (A)

CHAPTER 6
GRAPHIC EXPLANATIONS

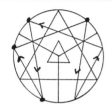

1 ÷ 7 = .142857

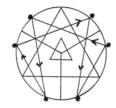

2 ÷ 7 = .285714

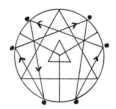

3 ÷ 7 = .428571

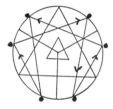

4 ÷ 7 = .571428

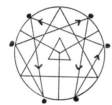

5 ÷ 7 = .714285

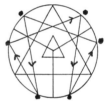

6 ÷ 7 = .857142

1 ÷ 7 =	1	4	2	8	5	7
	C	B	B	C	A	A
2 ÷ 7 =	2	8	5	7	1	4
	B	C	A	A	C	B
3 ÷ 7 =	4	2	8	5	7	1
	B	B	C	A	A	C
4 ÷ 7 =	5	7	1	4	2	8
	A	A	C	B	B	C
5 ÷ 7 =	7	1	4	2	8	5
	A	C	B	B	C	A
6 ÷ 7 =	8	5	7	1	4	2
	C	A	A	C	B	B

1 ÷ 7 = .142857 Diet CBBCAA

2 ÷ 7 = .285714 Medication BCAACB

3 ÷ 7 = .428571 Poison BBCAAC

4 ÷ 7 = .571428 Surgery AACBBC

5 ÷ 7 = .714285 Medication ACBBCA

6 ÷ 7 = .857142 Diet CAACBB

Summary of Restoration to Moral Balance Techniques

8
Diet: C to A positive
Med.: C to A positive
Poison: C to B negative
Surgery: C to A positive

1
Diet: C to B positive
Med.: C to B positive
Poison: C to A negative
Surgery: C to A positive

9o
Poison: C to C negative
Surgery: C to C positive

2
Diet: B to C positive
Med.: B to A positive
Poison: B to B negative
Surgery: B to C positive

4
Diet: B to B positive
Med.: B to C positive
Poison: B to C negative
Surgery: B to C positive

3o
Poison: A to A positive
Surgery: A to A negative

5
Diet: A to A positive
Med.: A to C positive
Poison: A to C negative
Surgery: A to B positive

7
Diet: A to C positive
Med.: A to B positive
Poison: A to A negative
Surgery: A to B positive

6o
Poison: A to A positive
Surgery: A to A
negative

Four Levels of Restoration to Moral Balance

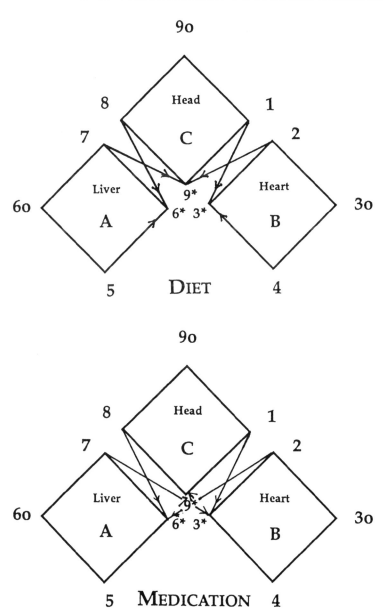

90

8   Head   1

7   C   2

Liver   9*   Heart

60   A   6* 3*   B   30

5   DIET   4

90

8   Head   1

7   C   2

Liver   9*   Heart

60   A   6* 3*   B   30

5   MEDICATION   4

FOUR LEVELS OF RESTORATION TO MORAL BALANCE

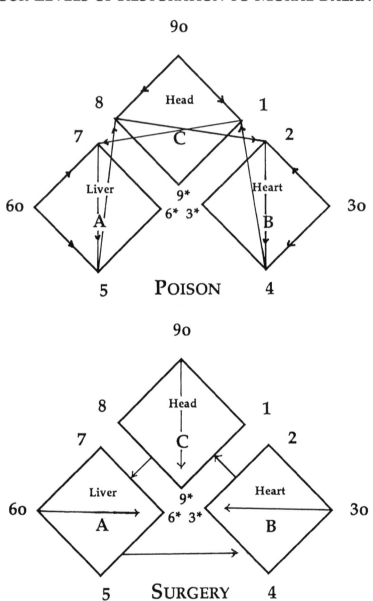

90

8 Head 1

7 C 2

Liver 9* Heart

60 A 6* 3* B 30

5 POISON 4

90

8 Head 1

7 C 2

Liver 9* Heart

60 A 6* 3* B 30

5 SURGERY 4

PARADIGM

NATURE

  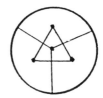

PROCESS

NUTURE

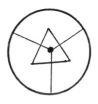 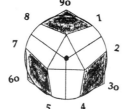 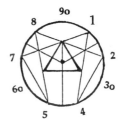

PROCEDURE

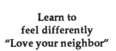

**Learn to
think differently
"Know yourself!"**

**Learn to
feel differently
"Love your neighbor"**

**Learn to
act differently
"Do good deeds"**

9o	6o	3o
Poison	Poison	Poison
Surgery	Surgery	Surgery

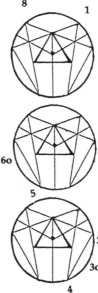

8
Diet
Medication
Poison
Surgery
1
Diet
Medication
Poison
Surgery
7
Diet
Medication
Poison
Surgery
5
Diet
Medication
Poison
Surgery
2
Diet
Medication
Poison
Surgery
4
Diet
Medication
Poison
Surgery

64 POSSIBLE MORAL BALANCES/IMBALANCES

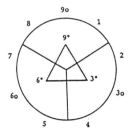
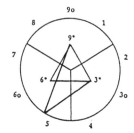

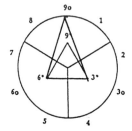
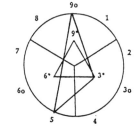

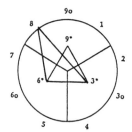
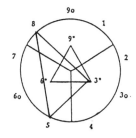

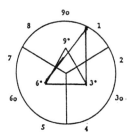
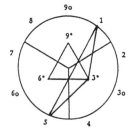

214

64 Possible Moral Balances/Imbalances

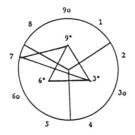
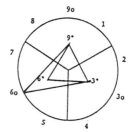

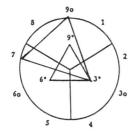
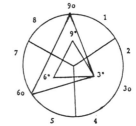

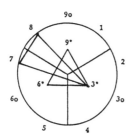
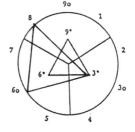

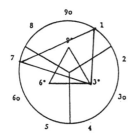
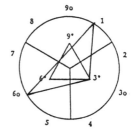

64 POSSIBLE MORAL BALANCES/IMBALANCES

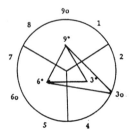
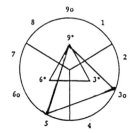

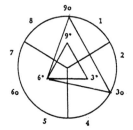
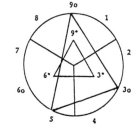

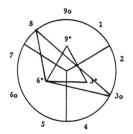
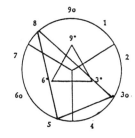

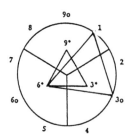
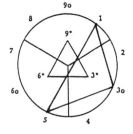

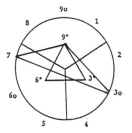
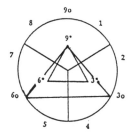

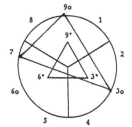
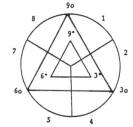

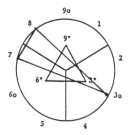
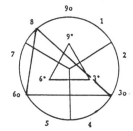

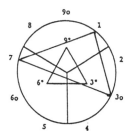
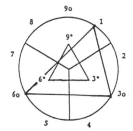

64 Possible Moral Balances/Imbalances

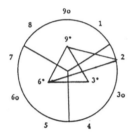

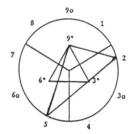

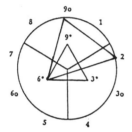

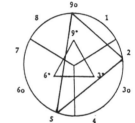

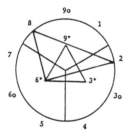

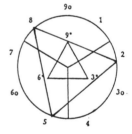

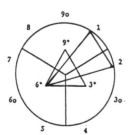

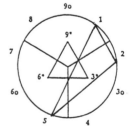

64 POSSIBLE MORAL BALANCES/IMBALANCES

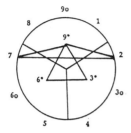
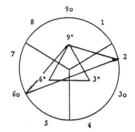

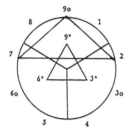
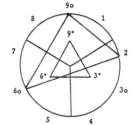

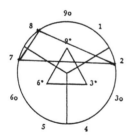
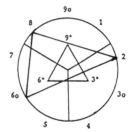

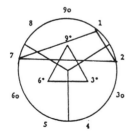
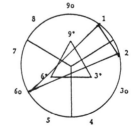

64 POSSIBLE MORAL BALANCES/IMBALANCES

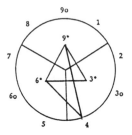
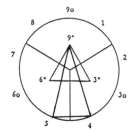

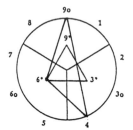
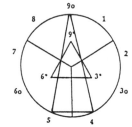

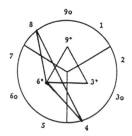
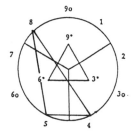

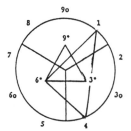
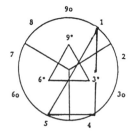

64 POSSIBLE MORAL BALANCES/IMBALANCES

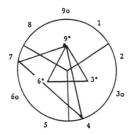

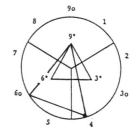

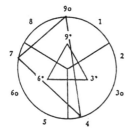

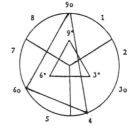

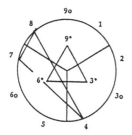

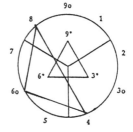

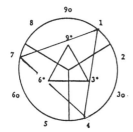

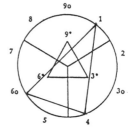

221

STAGE 1 (DIET)

IMBALANCE	BALANCE
1	COURAGE
8	TEMPERANCE
2	WISDOM
4	COURAGE
5	TEMPERANCE
7	WISDOM

STAGE 2 (MEDICATION)

IMBALANCE	BALANCE
1	COURAGE
8	TEMPERANCE
2	TEMPERANCE
4	WISDOM
5	WISDOM
7	COURAGE

STAGE 3 (POISON)

IMBALANCE	BALANCE
1	LUST
8	COWARDICE
2	ANGER
4	PRECONSCIOUSNESS
5	PRECONSCIOUSNESS
7	APATHY

STAGE 4 (SURGERY)

IMBALANCE	BALANCE
HYPOCRISY	AFFECT
MULTITHEISM	
COWARDICE	COGNITION
ANGER	
APATHY	BEHAVIOR
LUST	

Cognitive Techniques
Used with the Following Imbalances:

Diet
2 (B) to C positive
7 (A) to C positive

Medication
4 (B) to C positive
5 (A) to C positive

Poison
4 (A) to C negative
5 (A) to C negative
90 (C) to C negative

Surgery
2 (A) to C positive
4 (B) to C positive
90 (C) to C positive

Behavioral Techniques
Used with the Following Imbalances

Diet
4 (B) to B positive
1 (C) to B positive

Medication
7 (A) to B positive
1 (C) to B positive

Poison
2 (B) to B negative
3o (B) to B negative
8 (C) to B negative

Surgery
3o (B) to B positive
7 (A) to B positive

AFFECTIVE TECHNIQUES
USED WITH THE FOLLOWING IMBALANCES

DIET
5 (A) TO A POSITIVE
8 (C) TO A POSITIVE

MEDICATION
8 (C) TO A POSITIVE
2 (B) TO A POSITIVE

POISON
6O (A) TO A NEGATIVE
7 (A) TO A NEGATIVE
1 (C) TO A NEGATIVE

SURGERY
6O (A) TO A POSITIVE
7 (C) TO A POSITIVE
1 (C) TO A POSITIVE

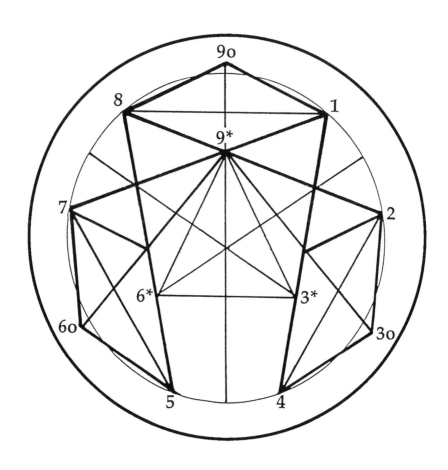

THE SIGN OF THE PRESENCE OF GOD (*WAJH ALLAH*)

This design was so named by the Naqshbandi Sufi Order in Central Asia. It is the origin of the Enneagram used in the West tody as a nine-point personality theory. The original design is to help the spiritual warrior attain moral healing thereby effecting the model of spiritual chivalry.

PART VII
MORAL HEALER'S DICTIONARY

The following dictionary has over three hundred entries of traits that cause moral imbalance. The keys to the restoration of moral balance based on the Sign of the Presence of God are given for each individual aspiring to moral goodness to be able to attain through continuous and strenuous self-examination.

Key to the Dictionary:

PsyType: The number is according to the Sign of the Presence of God. PsyTypes marked by an X are compound moral imbalances which are not dealt with in this handbook because the restoration to moral balance is beyond the self-help method of self-examination and needs the intervention of a Shaykh.

Effect: The effect of a PsyType is either positive or negative. Most of the positive effects given in the dictionary are the 99 Names and Qualities of God known to the spiritual warrior as the Most Beautiful Names. Only a person who has morally healed can manifest these qualities and, then, only through Divine Grace. They are qualities to aspire towards.

Those entries which have a positive effect which are not one of the 99 Most Beautiful Names (you will know because they have no Arabic equivalent nor do they have a Quality nor a Prayer) are a subcategory of one of the three traits of balance—wisdom, temperance or courage.

The levels of treatment of those entries which have a negative effect upon the self are described in detail in Part VI. The moral-seeker should find the number there, determine the level of entrenchment of the negative trait in self and then follow the procedure given to restore to moral balance. Ask a friend to help in the determination of the extent of entrenchment of a negative trait in yourself.

Quality: This entry is exclusive to the Divine Names and Qualities as positive traits and express its elemental quality (hot, cold, wet or dry) which is arrived at through letter symbolism of the Name or Quality in Arabic (see

Moral Healing Through the Most Beautiful Names, Volume 3 of *God's Will Be Done*).

Prayer: This entry is exclusive to the Divine Names and Qualities as positive traits. The prayers help the moral-seeker to advance on the spiritual path. The prayers have been translated from *Jawāhir al-khamsah* by Maulānā Mirzā Muḥammad Baiq Naqshbandī Dehlavī.

State: This indicates whether the entry is balanced or imbalanced and in which positive trait (wisdom, courage or temperance) it occurs.

Abaser, the (al-Khafid)

PsyType: 6*
Effect: Positive
Quality: Hot
Prayer: Fast for three days and on the fourth day, recite ya Khafid 70,000 times in a gathering and you should be free from harm by your enemy.

Able, the (al-Qadir)

PsyType: 9*
Effect: Positive
Quality: Cold
Prayer: Recite ya Qadir while washing each limb during the performance of the prescribed ablution and you should never fall into the grip of an oppressor and no enemy can harm you. If you face a difficulty and recite al-Qadir forty-one times, God should free you of that difficulty.

Abstinent

PsyType: 6*
State: Balanced in Temperance
Effect: Positive
Definition: Adorning yourself with moral deeds for the sake of the perfection of your innate nature and for the attainment of nearness to God.

All-Hearing, the (al-Sami)

PsyType: 9*
Effect: Positive
Quality: Hot
Prayer: Recite ya Sami 500 times after performing the noon prescribed prayer and God should hear your prayer and give you your desire.

All-Seeing, the (al-Basir)

PsyType: 9*
Effect: Positive
Quality: Hot
Prayer: Recite ya Basir 100 times after the Friday prescribed congregational prayer and God should give you esteem in the eyes of others.

Altruistic

PsyType: 3*
State: Balanced in Courage
Effect: Positive
Definition: Unselfish regard for or devotion to the welfare of others.

Anger, Inappropriate

PsyType: 4
State: Imbalanced in Courage
Effect: Negative
Cause: Overdevelopment of the instinct to preserve the individual.
Definition: A strong feeling of antagonism.

Anger, Lack of (see Cowardly)

PsyType: 2
State: Imbalanced in Courage
Effect: Negative
Cause: Underdevelopment of the instinct to preserve the individual.
Definition: Allowing others to debase and humiliate oneself and one's family.

Annoying

PsyType: 4
State: Imbalanced in Courage
Effect: Negative
Cause: Overdevelopment of the instinct to preserve the individual.
Definition: Implies a wearing on the nerves by persistent petty unpleasantness.

Anxiety

PsyType: 3o
State: Imbalanced in Courage

Effect: Negative

Cause: Undevelopment of the instinct to preserve the individual.

Definition: Painful or apprehensive uneasiness of mind usually over an impending or anticipated ill. It is to have fearful concern or interest and an abnormal and overwhelming sense of apprehension and fear marked by physiological signs such as sweating, tension, and increased pulse rate. It comes from being in doubt about the reality and nature of the threat and self-doubt in your capacity to cope with it.

Apathy in Regard to Food, Sex, Earning a Living

PsyType: 5

State: Imbalanced in Temperance

Effect: Negative

Cause: Underdevelopment of the instinct to preserve the species.

Definition: Lack of interest or concern with life. When you are so deprived in this world for neglecting to observe what is proper to daily living, this leads to the destruction of the human species.

Appraiser, the (al-Muhsi)

PsyType: 6*

Effect: Positive

Quality: Hot

Prayer: Recite ya Muhsi 100 times and one should receive ease on the Day of Judgment.

Arbiter, the (al-Hakam)

PsyType: 9*

Effect: Positive

Quality: Cold

Prayer: If one recites ya Hakam on Thursday night in the middle of the night so frequently and continuously that one loses consciousness and faints, one may come to know the hidden meanings in things.

Argumentative

PsyType: 4

State: Imbalanced in Courage

Effect: Negative

Cause: Overdevelopment of the instinct to preserve the individual.

Definition: Given to argument, disputations and being controversial; to argue with irritating persistence. It causes familiarity to disappear producing cleavage, mutual dislike and hostility while the order of the universe depends on familiarity and love.

Arrogant

PsyType: 4

State: Imbalanced in Courage

Effect: Negative

Cause: Overdevelopment of the instinct to preserve the individual.

Definition: When you think too highly of yourself, it is self-conceit. When you consider others as inferior, that is arrogance. Arrogance is a thick veil which hides the shortcomings from the self's view and prevents it from removing them and attaining perfection. It is a feeling or an impression of superiority manifested in an overbearing manner or presumptuous claims. Hadith: "Jesus said, 'Just as a plant grows in soft ground and not where the earth is rocky and hard, so also wisdom sprouts and grows in a heart which is humble and soft, not in the hard heart of the arrogant. Do you not see that a person who keeps his head high bashes it against the roof while one who holds his head low has the roof as his friend and shelter."

Aspiration
PsyType: 9*
State: Balanced in Wisdom
Effect: Positive
Definition: A strong desire to achieve something high or great.

Atheist (see Disbeliever)
PsyType: 9o
State: Imbalanced in Wisdom
Effect: Negative
Cause: Undevelopment of the instinct to preserve the true self.
Definition: Disbelief in the existence of a deity.

Avaricious (see Greedy)
PsyType: 7
State:Imbalance in Temperance
Effect: Negative
Cause: Overdevelopment in the instinct to preserve the species.
Definition: Greedy of gain; excessively acquisitive in seeking to hoard riches; having or showing a strong desire for material possession. It implies obsessive acquisitiveness especially of money and strong suggest stinginess.

Avenger, the (al-Muntaqim)
PsyType: 3*
Effect: Positive
Quality: Hot
Prayer: Repeat ya Muntaqim many times and you should be victorious against your enemy.

Aware, the (al-Khabir)
PsyType: 9*
Effect: Positive
Quality: Balanced in Hot/Cold

Prayer: Recite ya Khabir frequently and one should be quickly freed of a bad habit.

Backbite
PsyType: 6o
State: Balanced in Temperance
Effect: Positive
Cause: Undevelopment of the instinct to preserve the species.
Definition: To say mean or spiteful things about another person in their absence.

Bashful
PsyType: 2
State: Imbalanced in Courage
Effect: Negative
Cause: Underdevelopment of the instinct to preserve the individual.
Definition: Socially shy.

Beginner, the (al-Mubdi)
PsyType: 6*
Effect: Positive
Quality: Hot
Prayer: Repeat ya Mubdi and breathe towards someone who is in danger of losing something and they should be free of danger.

Begrudge
PsyType: 5
State: Imbalanced in
       Temperance
Effect: Negative
Cause: Underdevelopment in the instinct to preserve the species.
Definition: Grudgingly mean about spending or granting.

Bestower, the (al-Wahhab)
PsyType: 3*
Effect: Positive
Quality: Hot
Prayer: Repeat ya Wahhab

seven times at midnight after suppli-
cation and your appeal should be
answered. If you have a desire or have
been captured by an enemy or cannot
earn enough, for three or seven nights,
repeat ya Wahhab 100 times after a
two-cycle midnight prayer with ablution and God should bless your needs.

Boastfulness

PsyType: 4
State: Imbalanced in Courage
Effect: Negative
Cause: Overdevelopment of the
instinct to preserve the individual.
Definition: Taking pride in
things external to yourself. Hadith:
"Do not bring your ancestry to me;
bring me your own actions."

Break Ties with Your Family

PsyType: X
Effect: Negative
Definition: To refuse to contact
one's family.
Discussion: This negative trait is
caused by hostility, vengefulness, jealousy, or miserliness. It prevents socia-
bility, hospitality and friendliness.

Brutal (see Cruel)

PsyType: X
Effect: Negative
Definition: Grossly ruthless or
unfeeling.

Callous (see Cruel)

PsyType: X
Effect: Negative
Definition: Feeling no emotion, it
is difficult to get rid of this negative
trait because cruelty and callousness
are traits which sink into one's character and become chronic. It is best to
avoid all cruel actions. Make an effort

to share in the sufferings and difficulties of others and to consider their
problems your own until compassion
becomes a permanent part of your
character.

Certainty

PsyType: 9*
State: Balanced in Wisdom
Imbalance: C
Effect: Positive
Definition: Opposite of ignorance, perplexity and doubt. Certainty
is lasting, certain conviction which
being in accordance with reality cannot be shaken by doubts however
strong. To have certainty is to rely on
God in all one's affairs knowing,
"There is no power except that it be
derived from God." Humility before
God, both inwardly and outwardly, at
all times and under all circumstances
is a sign of certainty of faith. Hadith:
"Certainty is complete belief."

Cheerful

PsyType: 6*
State: Balanced in Temperance
Effect: Positive
Definition: Full of good spirits.

Clarity of Mind

PsyType: 9*
State:Balanced in Wisdom
Effect: Positive
Definition: You realize an apti-
tude for extracting the desired result
without experiencing any agitation or
confusion.

Clement, the (al-Ra'uf)

PsyType: 3*
Effect: Positive
Quality: Hot
Prayer: Repeat ya Ra'uf fre-

quently and one should be blessed by God and His people.

Collected

> PsyType: 3*
> State: Balanced in Courage
> Effect: Positive
> Definition: Self's constancy in its own stability at the moment of entering upon difficulties and dangers that it give no room to fear and no rise to unsteady impulses.

Compassionate, the (al-Rahim)

> PsyType: 3*
> Effect: Positive
> Quality: Balanced in Hot/Cold
> Prayer: Repeat 100 times after each dawn prescribed prayer and everyone should become friendly towards you.

Compeller, the (al-Jabbar)

> PsyType: 6*
> Effect: Positive
> Quality: Balanced in Hot/Cold
> Prayer: Repeat ya Jabbar twenty-one times frequently and you should not be compelled to do anything against your wishes nor should you be exposed to violence or hardship.

Complacent

> PsyType: 5
> State: Imbalanced in
>   Temperance
> Effect: Negative
> Cause: Underdevelopment of the instinct to preserve the species.
> Definition: Self-satisfaction accompanied by unawareness of actual dangers or deficiencies.

Conceal the Truth

> PsyType: 4
> State: Imbalanced in Courage

Effect: Negative
Cause: Overdevelopment of instinct to preserve the individual.
> Definition: Misrepresentation and concealment of the truth, the negative trait of concealing the truth is caused by fanaticism, cowardice or fear. It causes you to deviate from the Straight Path and it brings moral degeneration.

Concealer of Faults, the (al-Ghafur)

> PsyType: 3*
> Effect: Positive
> Quality: Balanced in Hot/Cold
> Prayer: Whenever you suffer from a headache, fever or temporary despair and despondency, you should recite ya Ghafur continuously and you may be relieved of your ailment.

Conceited

> PsyType: 4
> State: Imbalanced in Courage
> Effect: Negative
> Cause: Overdevelopment of the instinct to preserve the individual.
> Definition: Excessive appreciation of one's own worth or virtue. This may be caused by arrogance, forgetfulness, negligence of your faults, falling of worth of your deeds in the eyes of people and God, absence of gratitude for God's blessings and thus risking their loss; failure to ask questions about the things of which one is ignorant and therefore remaining in ignorance; holding and proclaiming of incorrect and unfounded opinions being favored with knowledge, devotion, piety, faith, courage, generosity, patience, and intelligence and devel-

oping conceit because of it. Every human being is in love with his or her 'self' according to Alrazes. Therefore, you see only your positive qualities and overlook your negative ones. This develops into conceit especially if others support this in you. You never, then, seek to improve or inquire from others about the quality for which you are conceited. Your conceit becomes an obstacle to knowledge and action. Hadith: "Even if you do not commit any sins, I fear you may fall into something which is worse: conceit! conceit!" And, "Do not boast of your riches, vigor and elegance since the first can be taken away by thieves and the other two can vanish in the signs of the appearance of fever."

Conjecture

PsyType: 1
State: Imbalanced in Wisdom
Effect: Negative
Cause: Overdevelopment of the instinct to preserve the true self.

Definition: Inference from defective or presumptive evidence; a conclusion deducted by surmise and guess work.

Consciousness

PsyType: 9*
State: Balanced in Wisdom
Effect: Positive
Definition: The state of being aware to some extent of one's sensations, emotions, volition, and thoughts.

Constant

PsyType: 9*
State: Balanced in Wisdom

Effect: Positive
Definition: Marked by firm, steadfast resolution or faithfulness.

Constrictor, the (al-Qabid)

PsyType: 6*
State: Balanced in Temperance
Effect: Positive
Quality: Hot
Prayer: For forty days write ya Qabid on a piece of bread and one should be safe from the punishment of the grave.

Contemplative

PsyType: 9*
State: Balanced in Wisdom
Effect: Positive
Definition:Concentration on spiritual things as a form of private devotion.

Contemptuous

PsyType: 1
State: Imbalanced in Wisdom
Effect: Negative
Cause: Overdevelopment of the instinct to preserve the true self.

Definition: The act of despising another. It is a negative trait, in general, but in particular when used against one's parents (17:23), orphans (93:90 or the needy (93:10).

Content

PsyType: 9*
State: Balanced in Wisdom
Effect: Positive
Definition: It is to control your desires so as to be content with having the basic necessities of life. If you attain this positive trait, you will be able to live as a free human being because you will be immune from the negative traits of affluence in this

world and the consequent punishment in the Hereafter.

Cool

PsyType: 3*
State: Balanced in Courage
Effect: Positive
Definition: You do not act with haste nor are you overcome by anger.

Counsel to the Positive

PsyType: 9*
State: Balanced in Wisdom
Effect: Positive
Definition: Guide the self and others to the positive.

Courage

PsyType: 3*
State: Balanced in Courage
Effect: Positive
Definition: Moderate state of the avoidance of harm/pain and the middle way between cowardice and recklessness. Courage is a virtue only when practiced in the right circumstances and in the right way. Thus, it is not a strength or mercy which is commendable in itself. Circumstances will determine the appropriate amount of strength or mercy to show depending upon what reason determines. Courage is to struggle with the ego and in doing so, to awaken the spirit within through developing a sense of humility towards others.

Covetous (see Greedy)

PsyType: 7
State: Imbalanced in
    Temperance
Effect: Negative
Cause: Overdevelopment of the instinct to preserve the species.
Definition: Marked by inordinate desire for wealth or possessions or for another's possessions.

Cowardly

PsyType: 2
State: Imbalanced in Courage
Effect: Negative
Cause: Underdevelopment of the instinct to preserve the individual.
Definition: Quiescence of the self when it should be agitated and an absence of the passion for revenge. This negative trait may be caused by laziness and love of ease or feelings of inferiority, irresolution, melancholy, and a lack of self-confidence. It results in humiliation and an unfortunate life in being at the mercy of one's relatives or those with whom you have to deal. It is to become subservient to everyone, accepting every kind of humiliation or wrong. It is to endure all sorts of offensive remarks in regard to yourself, your relatives or your family. It can be accompanied by certain types of perversion such as light-mindedness, want of constancy in relationships, indolence and love of ease. The Quran says that to show weakness in face of difficulties or to lose heart (8:46); to be weak in will (3:146); to be faint-hearted (47:35); to despair (57:23); to be afraid of other people (4:77); or to be afraid of satan (3:175) are negative traits.

Crafty (see Cunning)

PsyType: 1
State: Imbalanced in Wisdom
Effect: Negative
Cause: Overdevelopment of the instinct to preserve the true self.
Definition: Implies cleverness

and subtlety of method.Other synonyms include: slyness which implies furtiveness, lack of candor, and skill in concealing one's aims and methods; cunning suggests the inventive use of sometimes limited intelligence in overreaching or circumventing; crafty implies cleverness and subtlety of method; tricky is more likely to suggest shiftiness and unreliability than skill in deception; foxy implies a shrewd and wary craftiness usually involving devious dealing; artful implies alluring indirectness in dealing and often connotes sophistication or cleverness.

Creator of the Beneficial, the

(al-Nafi)

PsyType: 6*
Effect: Positive
Quality: Hot
Prayer: Repeat ya Nafi for four days as many times as one can and one should be able to avoid harm.

Creator of the Harmful, the

(al-Darr)

PsyType: 6*
Effect: Positive
Quality: Hot
Prayer: If you have been in the same state or condition for a long time and want to get into better state, if you repeat ya Darr 100 times on Thursday nights, you should grow closer to God.

Creator, the (al-Khaliq)

PsyType: 6*
Effect: Positive
Quality: Cold
Prayer: Recite ya Khaliq frequently at night and God may help

you act for His sake.

Cruel

PsyType: X
Effect: Negative
Definition: Disposed to inflict pain or suffering; devoid of humane feelings. Causing or conducive to injury, grief, or pain.

Cunning

PsyType: 1
State: Imbalanced in Wisdom
Effect: Negative
Cause: Overdevelopment of the instinct to preserve the true self.

Definition: Characterized by wiliness and trickery. The intellect is so immersed in meticulous examination that one loses one's sense of balance. It is an overdevelopment of mental activity that takes you further and further away from reality and causes you to be bogged down in doubt and indecision.

Curser

PsyType: X
Effect: Negative
Definition: A prayer for injury to come upon another; to use profanity against someone.

Debasement of Aspiration

PsyType: 7
State: Imbalanced in Temperance
Effect: Negative
Cause: Overdevelopment of the instinct to preserve the species.

Definition: Deterioration of aspiration; loss of worth, value or dignity. Debase implies a loss of position, worth, value or dignity. Synonyms include: deprave which implies moral deterioration by evil thoughts or influences; corrupt which implies loss of soundness, purity or integrity; debauch which implies debasing through sensual indulgences; pervert which implies a twisting or distorting from what is natural or normal.

Deceitful

PsyType: 1
State: Imbalanced in Wisdom
Effect: Negative
Cause: Overdevelopment of the instinct to reason.

Definition: To cause to accept as true or valid what is false or invalid; to give a false impression.

Delighting in the Misfortune of Others

PsyType: 3o
State: Imbalanced in Courage
Effect: Negative
Cause: Undevelopment in the instinct to preserve the individual.

Definition: To be happy when others suffer misfortune.

Denial

PsyType: 9o
State: Imbalanced in Wisdom
Imbalance: C
Effect: Negative
Cause: Undevelopment of the instinct to reason.

Definition: Refusal to admit the truth or reality; refusal to acknowledge a person or thing.

Derision

PsyType: 4
State: Imbalanced in Courage
Effect: Negative
Cause: Overdevelopment of the instinct to preserve the individual.

Definition: You begin to accept ridicule and then expose yourself to even greater ridicule in order to arouse laughter of others and to receive a little of their favor.

Deserter

PsyType: 2
State: Imbalanced in Courage
Effect: Negative
Cause: Underdevelopment of the instinct to preserve the individual.

Definition: Abandonment without consent or legal justification of a person, post or relationship and the associated duties and obligations.

Despair

PsyType: 5
State:Imbalanced in Temperance
Effect: Negative
Cause: Underdevelopment of the instinct to preserve the species.

Definition: To lose all hope or confidence.

Dignity, Lack of a Sense of

PsyType: 2
State: Imbalanced in Courage
Effect: Negative
Cause: Underdevelopment of the instinct to preserve the individual.

Definition: Lack of enough attention and failure to take care of matters which need attention and care like your faith, honor, children and property.

Disbeliever

PsyType: 9o
State: Imbalanced in Wisdom
Effect: Negative
Cause: Undevelopment of the instinct to reason.

Definition: To "cover over the truth" by denying the existence of God.

Disclosing People's Secrets

    PsyType: X
    Effect: Negative
    Definition: To reveal people's secrets which have been entrusted to you.

Discord, Causing

    PsyType: X
    Effect: Negative
    Definition: Implies an intrinsic or essential lack of harmony. Causing discord, disharmony, disorder or disunity (2:191, 192, 205; 7:85; 11:85) stands against unity. It is the ego that incites one to discord (7:200; 41:36) in its lack of wisdom (59:14). Synonyms include: strife which emphasizes a struggle for superiority rather than the incongruity or incompatibility of the persons or things involved; conflict which stresses the action of forces in opposition but in static applications implies an irreconcilability as of duties or desires; contention which applies to strife or competition that shows itself in quarreling, disputing or controversy; dissension which implies strife or discord and stresses a division into factions; and variance which implies a clash between persons or things owing to a difference in nature, opinion or interest.

Dishonorer, the (al-Mudhill)

    PsyType: 6*
    Effect: Positive
    Quality: Hot
    Prayer: Recite ya Mudhill seven-

ty-five times when you sense harm from a jealous person and you should be protected by God. If you go to prostration and say, "O God save me from the oppression of so and so..." you should be saved.

Dissimulation

    PsyType: 5
    State: Imbalanced in Temperance
    Effect: Negative
    Cause: Underdevelopment of the instinct to preserve the species.
    Definition: Hiding under a false appearance.

Doubtful

    PsyType: 1
    State: Imbalanced in Wisdom
    Effect: Negative
    Cause: Overdevelopment of the instinct to reason.
    Definition: To lack confidence in something or someone, to be continuously in a state of doubt is to be mistrustful. It also means uncertainty of belief or opinion that often interferes with decision-making.

Drawing Closer to God

    PsyType: 9*
    State: Balanced in Wisdom
    Effect: Positive
    Definition: Consciously choosing to empty self of everything but the desire to grow closer to God.

Earnings, Illegitimate

    PsyType: 7
    State: Balanced in Temperance
    Effect: Negative
    Cause: Overdevelopment of the instinct to preserve the species.
    Definition: Amassing of wealth in

an illegitimate manner. Hadith: "Whoever lives on legitimate earnings for forty days, God shall enlighten his heart and cause springs of wisdom to emanate from his heart flowing to his tongue."

Ease of Learning

PsyType: 9*
State: **Balanced in Wisdom**
Effect: **Positive**
Definition: You acquire a sharpness of vision so as to direct yourself wholly towards the desired object without the hindrance of random thoughts.

Endurance

PsyType: 3*
State: **Balanced in Courage**
Effect: **Positive**
Definition: The ability to withstand hardship, adversity or stress.

Enmity

PsyType: 4
State: **Imbalanced in Courage**
Effect: **Negative**
Cause: Overdevelopment of the instinct to preserve the individual.
Definition: It is deep-seated dislike or ill will which may be open or concealed. When you repress your anger and the repression is ineffective because your sense of anger is not satisfied or expressed, it returns to yourself, is constricted and becomes enmity. You may develop envy and be happy at another's misfortune. At the lest serious level, when your mind is burdened with some enmity against another person, you cease to favor him, to stand beside him in his need, to associate with him, and to encourage him to good. When anger is repressed or suppressed, you become jealous and sever relations with someone against whom your enmity is directed. This may result in physical assault, spreading of lies, backbiting, slander, the divulging of secrets, and so forth. If you show your enmity, this may develop into outright hostility resulting in confrontation, fighting, cursing, and name-calling.

Enricher, the (al-Mughni)

PsyType: 3*
Effect: **Positive**
Quality: **Hot**
Prayer: Recite ya Mughni 1000 times every Friday and one should become self-sufficient.

Envious

PsyType: 60
State:Imbalanced in Temperance
Effect: **Positive**
Cause: Undevelopment of the instinct to preserve the individual.
Definition: Sometimes envy is considered to be a compound of ignorance and wanting more or greed. Results in depression. It differs from emulation or longing to acquire a perfection or a desired object without any wish for its removal from the other person.

Equitable, the (al-Muqsit)

PsyType: 6*
Effect: **Positive**
Quality: **Balanced in Hot/Cold**
Prayer: Repeat ya Muqsit 100 times and you should be free from the harm of your ego and you should attain your purpose.

Eternal, the (al-Samad)
PsyType: 9*
Effect: Positive
Quality: Hot
Prayer: Repeat ya Samad 1000
times and you may come to know the
hidden meaning of things. If you
recite ya Samad at dawn or in the middle of the night while in prostration
115 times, you should never fall into
the grip of an oppressor.

Everlasting, the (al-Baqi)
PsyType: 9*
Effect: Positive
Quality: Hot
Prayer: Recite ya Baqi on
Thursday night and you should be free
of difficulties.

Exalted, the (al-Muta'ali)
PsyType: 9*
Effect: Positive
Quality: Hot
Prayer: Repeat ya Muta'ali fre-
quently and you should gain the
benevolence of God and difficulties
should ease.

Exalter, the (al-Rafi)
PsyType: 6*
Effect: Positive
Quality: Balanced in Hot/Cold
Prayer: Recite ya Rafi 100 times
on Thursday and Sunday night and
you should attain a higher sense of
honor, richness and merit.

Excessive Speech
PsyType: 1
State: Imbalanced in Wisdom
Effect: Negative
Cause: Overdevelopment of the
instinct to preserve the true self.
Definition: Talking too much.

Expander, the (al-Basit)
PsyType: 6*
Effect: Positive
Quality: Balanced in Hot/Cold
Prayer: Recite ya Basit ten times
during the dawn prescribed prayer
with open hands, palms up and then
rub your face with your hands and you
should be freed of the need of others.

Extravagant (see Prodigal)
PsyType: 7
State: Imbalanced in
         Temperance
Effect: Negative
Cause: Overdevelopment of the
instinct to preserve the species.
Definition: Exceeding the limits
of reason or necessity; lacking in
moderation, balance, and restraint;
excessively elaborate.

Faint-hearted (see Cowardly)
PsyType: 2
State: Imbalanced in Courage
Imbalance: B
Effect: Negative
Cause: Underdevelopment of
the instinct to preserve the individual.
Definition: Lacking courage or
resolution.

Faith, the Giver of (al-Mu'min)
PsyType: 3*
Effect: Positive
Quality: Hot
Prayer: Recite ya Mu'min fre-
quently and you should be freed from
the harm of your false self.

False Promises, Make (see Deceit)
PsyType: 1
State: Imbalanced in Wisdom

Effect: Negative
Cause: Overdevelopment of the instinct to reason.
Definition: Not keeping one's promises.

Fanatic

PsyType: 4
State: Imbalance in Courage
Effect: Negative
Cause: Overdevelopment of the instinct to preserve the individual.

Definition: Marked by excessive enthusiasm and often intense uncritical devotion, to have this negative trait it to be prejudiced in regard to your religious beliefs, nation, tribe, family or other such things. It may be manifested through your speech or actions. Hadith: "Whoever has the least amount of fanaticism in his heart shall be raised by God on the Day of Resurrection together with the pagan Arabs of pre-Islamic times."

Fatalistic

PsyType: 9o
State: Imbalanced in Wisdom
Effect: Negative
Cause: Undevelopment of the instinct to reason.

Definition: Belief that events are fixed in advance for all time in such a manner that human beings are powerless to change them.

Fear

PsyType: 3o
State: Imbalanced in Courage
Effect: Negative
Cause: Undevelopment of the instinct to preserve the individual.

Definition: Unpleasant and often strong emotion caused by anticipation or awareness of danger; anxious concern. When fear of other than God develops from a combination of both underdevelopment and overdevelopment of courage, you pass beyond tormenting people and begin to torment tongue-tied beasts and inanimate objects like furnishings. You seek relief by trying to strike donkeys and cows or to kill pigeons and cats or to break tools. Synonyms include: dread which adds the intense reluctance to face or meet a person or situation and suggests aversion as well as anxiety; fright which implies the shock of sudden, startling fear; alarm which suggests a sudden and intense awareness of an immediate danger; panic which implies unreasoning and overmastering of fear causing hysterical activity; terror which implies the most extreme degree of fear; trepidation adds to dread the implication of timidity, trembling and hesitation.

Fear of Death

PsyType: 3o
State: Imbalanced in Courage
Effect: Negative
Cause: Undevelopment of the instinct to preserve the individual.

Definition: Fear of what happens to you after you die.

Fear of Other than God

PsyType: 3o
State: Imbalanced in Courage
Effect: Negative
Cause: Undevelopment of the instinct to preserve the individual.

Definition: Fear is of two kinds: the first, fear of God and fear of wrongdoings and punishment. This kind of fear is praiseworthy and leads the human being to perfection. The second kind is depravity of your natural disposition of avoidance of harm/pain or instinct to preserve the individual.

Fearful of God

PsyType: 6*
State: Balanced in Temperance
Effect: Positive
Definition: To be pious and god-fearing.

Firm, the (al-Matin)

PsyType: 9*
Effect: Positive
Quality: Hot
Prayer: Recite ya Matin frequently if you have troubles and your troubles should disappear.

First, the (al-Awwal)

PsyType: 9*
Effect: Positive
Quality: Hot
Prayer: Recite ya Awwal forty times on Thursday nights and your needs should be fulfilled.

Flawless, the (al-Salam)

PsyType: 9*
Effect: Positive
Quality: Hot
Prayer: Recite ya Salam 110 times to a sick person and the person may regain their health.

Foolhardiness (see Recklessness)

PsyType: 4
State: Imbalanced in Courage
Effect: Negative
Cause: Overdevelopment of the instinct to preserve the individual.

Definition: Reckless entrance into dangerous and deadly situations despite the warnings of reason and religion. "*And cast not yourselves by your own hands into destruction...*" (2:195).

Foolish

PsyType: 1
State: **Imbalanced in Wisdom**
Effect: **Negative**
Cause: Overdevelopment of the instinct to reason.
Definition: Absurd or ridiculous behavior or idea.

Forebearing, the (al-Halim)

PsyType: 3*
Effect: Positive
Quality: Balanced in Hot/Cold
Prayer: Write ya Halim on a piece of paper and put the paper wherever one plants a seed to preserve the seed from harm, disaster or calamity.

Forgiver, the (al-Ghaffar)

PsyType: 3*
Effect: Positive
Quality: Balanced in Hot/Cold
Prayer: Recite ya Ghaffar 100 times after the Friday prescribed congregational prayer and your sins should be forgiven.

Fortitude

PsyType: 3*
State: **Balanced in Wisdom**
Effect: Positive
Definition: Strength of character that enables you to encounter danger or bear pain and adversity with courage.

Free

PsyType: 6*
State:Balanced in Temperance

Effect: Positive

Definition: Permanent removal from whatever binds, confines, entangles, or oppresses.

Friend, the (al-Wali)

PsyType: 3*

Effect: Positive

Quality: Hot

Prayer: Recite ya Wali frequently and you may become a Friend of God.

Friendly (see Friend)

PsyType: 3*

State: Balanced in Courage

Effect: Positive

Definition: Showing kindly interest and goodwill towards one's friends. Hadith: "When God loves one of His servants, He blesses him (or her) with the trait of friendliness and whoever lacks this trait, lacks other blessings as well."

Gatherer, the (al-Jami)

PsyType: 6*

Effect: Positive

Quality: Balanced in Hot/Cold

Prayer: Repeat ya Jami frequently to find things lost.

Generous, the (al-Karim)

PsyType: 3*

Effect: Positive

Quality: Balanced in Hot/Cold

Prayer: Recite ya Karim frequently and you should have esteem in this world.

Gentle

PsyType: 3*

State: Balanced in Courage

Effect: Positive

Definition: It is to restrain yourself from inappropriate anger. Anger is a natural trait and needed but it needs to be refined and developing gentleness helps refine anger.

Glorious, the (al-Majid)

PsyType: 9*

Effect: Positive

Quality: Balanced in Cold/Hot

Prayer: Recite ya Majid frequently and you should gain glory.

Gluttonous

PsyType: 7

State: Imbalanced in Temperance

Effect: Negative

Cause: Overdevelopment of the instinct to preserve the species.

Definition: Excess in eating or drinking. This is considered to be the first negative trait from which you should be freed.

Good Appearance

PsyType: 6*

State: Balanced in Courage

Effect: Positive

Definition: The desire of necessary attire without any frivolity.

Good (see Source of All Goodness)

PsyType: 9*

State: Balanced in Wisdom

Effect: Positive

Definition: Conforming to the moral order of the universe.

Goodness, the Source of All (al-Barr)

PsyType: 9*

Effect: Positive

Quality: Balanced in Hot/Cold

Prayer: Repeat ya Barr frequently and you should be blessed and free from misfortune.

Governor, the (al-Wali)

PsyType: 6*
Effect: Positive
Quality: Hot
Prayer: Repeat ya Wali in your home and it should be free from danger.

Great, the (al-Kabir)

PsyType: 9*
Effect: Positive
Quality: Balanced in Hot/Cold
Prayer: Repeat ya Kabir 100 times frequently and you should develop esteem and respect among people.

Greedy

PsyType: 7
State: Imbalanced in Temperance
Effect: Negative
Cause: Overdevelopment of the instinct to preserve the species.

Definition: Exceeding what is necessary. It includes selfishness and often suggests unfair or ruthless means to get what you want. It is to be dissatisfied with whatever you have and to yearn for yet more. It is not limited to worldly possessions but includes over indulgence in food, sex and so forth. Hadith: "The greedy man in his love of the world is like a silkworm. The more you wrap yourself in your cocoon, the less chance you have of escaping from it until you finally die of grief."

Grieving

PsyType: 60
State: Imbalanced in Temperance

Effect: Positive
Cause: Undevelopment of the instinct to preserve the species.

Definition: Deep distress caused by or as if by bereavement.

Guardian, the (al-Muhaymin)

PsyType: 3*
Effect: Positive
Quality: Hot
Prayer: Recite ya Muhaymin after the prescribed ablution 115 times and your inner being may be illuminated.

Guide, the (al-Hadi)

PsyType: 3*
Effect: Positive
Quality: Hot
Prayer: Repeat ya Hadi frequently and you should gain spiritual knowledge.

Hard-hearted

PsyType: 4
State: Imbalanced in Courage
Effect: Negative
Cause: Overdevelopment of the instinct to preserve the individual

Definition: Lacking in sympathetic understanding; unfeeling; pitiless.

Harsh

PsyType: 4
State: Imbalanced in Courage
Effect: Negative
Cause: Overdevelopment of the instinct to preserve the individual.

Definition: Unduly exacting; severe.

Hasty

PsyType: 4
State: Imbalanced in Courage
Effect: Negative

Cause: Overdevelopment of the instinct to preserve the individual.

Definition: Acting in a hurry and usually superficially. It shows a weakness of character and possible inferiority complex.

Hatred

> **PsyType:** X
> **Imbalance:** X
> **Effect:** Negative
> **Definition:** Implies an emotional aversion often coupled with enmity or malice. Synonyms include: detest which suggests violent antipathy; abhor which implies a deep, often shuddering repugnance; abominate which suggests a strong detestation and often moral condemnation; loathe which implies utter disgust and intolerance.

Hidden, the (al-Batin)

> **PsyType:** 9*
> **Effect:** Positive
> **Quality:** Hot
> **Prayer:** Recite ya Batin twenty-two times each day and you may see the truth in things.

Highest, the (al-Ali)

> **PsyType:** 9*
> **Effect:** Positive
> **Quality:** Cold
> **Prayer:** If your faith is low and you repeat ya 'Ali frequently, your faith should be raised and your destiny opened.

Hoard

> **PsyType:** 7
> **State:** Temperance
> **Effect:** Negative
> **Cause:** Overdevelopment
> **Definition:** To hide a supply of

something or store up; to keep to oneself.

Holy, the (al-Quddus)

> **PsyType:** 9*
> **Effect:** Positive
> **Quality:** Cold
> **Prayer:** If you recite ya Quddus each day at sunset, your heart may expand.

Honorer, the (al-Muizz)

> **PsyType:** 6*
> **Effect:** Positive
> **Quality:** Cold
> **Prayer:** If you repeat ya Muizz 140 times after the evening prescribed prayer on Sunday and Thursday night, you should develop dignity in the eyes of others and fear no one but God.

Hopeful

> **PsyType:** 6*
> **State: Balanced in Temperance**
> **Effect:** Positive
> **Definition:** To cherish a desire with the expectation of fulfillment.

Hostile

> **PsyType:** 4
> **State:** **Imbalanced in Courage**
> **Effect:** Negative
> **Cause:** Overdevelopment of the instinct to preserve the individual.
> **Definition:** Conflict, opposition or resistance in thought or principle, enmity.

Humility

> **PsyType:** 3*
> **State:** **Balanced in Courage**
> **Effect:** Positive
> **Definition:** Implies self-abasement.

Hypocrite

> **PsyType:** 1

State: **Imbalanced in Wisdom**
Effect: **Negative**
Cause: Overdevelopment of the instinct to reason.

Definition: Pretending to be what you are not or to believe what you are not; the false assumption of an appearance of virtue or religion. It is to say with your tongue what is not in your heart (2:167; 4:81; 47:11). It is to be distracted in mind being sincerely neither for one group nor for another (4:143). Hypocrites are liars (59:11; 3:188) and expect praise for what they never do. They compete with each other in sin and rancor (5:65).

Identification

PsyType: **9o**
State: **Imbalanced in Wisdom**
Effect: **Negative**
Cause: Undevelopment of the instinct to reason.

Definition: Psychological orientation of yourself in regard to something (as a person or group) with a resulting feeling or process where without awareness of what you are doing, you model the thoughts, feelings and actions after those of an external object that has been incorporated in a mental image.

Ignorant

PsyType: **8**
State: **Imbalanced in Wisdom**
Effect: **Negative**
Cause: Underdevelopment of the instinct to reason.

Definition: General condition or lack of knowledge of a particular thing.

Ill-tempered

PsyType: **4**
State: **Imbalanced in Courage**
Effect: **Negative**
Cause: Overdevelopment of the instinct to preserve the individual.

Definition: Ill-natured, quarrelsome. Hadith: "Ill-temper ruins good works just as vinegar ruins honey."

Impassive (see Apathy)

PsyType: **5**
State: **Imbalanced in Temperance**
Effect: **Negative**
Cause: Underdevelopment of the instinct to preserve the species.

Definition: Giving no sign of feeling or emotion.

Impatient

PsyType: **4**
State: **Imbalanced in Courage**
Effect: **Negative**
Cause: Overdevelopment of the instinct to preserve the individual.

Definition: Not patient; restless; short of temper especially under irritation, delay or opposition.

Impudent

PsyType: **7**
State: **Imbalanced in Temperance**
Effect: **Negative**
Cause: Overdevelopment of the instinct to preserve the individual.

Definition: Lacking modesty; disregard of others.

Incomparable, the (al-Aziz)

PsyType: **9***
Effect: **Positive**
Quality: **Cold**
Prayer: If you recite ya 'Aziz for forty days between the prescribed

and recommended dawn prayer, you should not be needy.

Inconstancy in Affairs
PsyType: 9o
State: Imbalanced in Wisdom
Effect: Negative
Cause: Undevelopment of the instinct to reason.
Definition: Lacking firmness or steadiness as in purpose or devotion. Synonyms include: inconstant which implies an incapacity for steadiness and an inherent tendency to change; fickle which suggests unreliability because of perverse changeability and incapacity for steadfastness; capricious which suggests motivation by sudden whim or fancy and stresses unpredictability; mercurial which implies rapid changeability in mood; and unstable which implies an incapacity for remaining in a field position or steady course and applies especially to emotional imbalance.

Indifferent (see Apathy)
PsyType: 5
Effect: Negative
Cause: Underdevelopment of the instinct to preserve the species.
Definition: Marked by no special liking for or dislike of something and by a lack of interest, enthusiasm or concern for something.

Ingratitude
PsyType: X
Imbalance: X
Effect: Negative
Definition: Ungratefulness; forgetfulness or poor return for kindness received. Quran: *"If you are thankful, I will give you more but if you are ungrateful, My punishment is surely terrible"* (14:7); *"God has struck a similitude: A city that was secure and well content, its provision coming to it in abundance from every place, then it was unthankful for God's blessings. God let it taste the garment of hunger and fear for the things that they were working"* (16:112).

Inheritor, the (al-Warith)
PsyType: 6*
Effect: Positive
Quality: Balanced in Hot/Cold
Prayer: Recite ya Warith 100 times at sunrise and you should be free of difficulties. If you recite it often, your work should be fulfilled.

Injustice, Toleration of
PsyType: 3o
State: Imbalanced in Courage
Effect: Negative
Cause: Undevelopment of the instinct to preserve the individual.
Definition: Tolerating any act that involves unfairness or violation of one's rights.

Intellection, Excellence of
PsyType: 9*
State: Balanced in Wisdom
Effect: Positive

Intrepid (see Bold)
PsyType: 3*
State: Balanced in Courage
Effect: Positive
Definition: Confidence of the self in facing death, when necessary without fear. It corresponds to courage in the sense of bravery in the battlefield.

Introjection
PsyType: 9o

State: **Imbalanced in Wisdom**
Effect: **Negative**
Cause: Undevelopment of the instinct to reason.

Definition: To incorporate attitudes or ideas into your personality without the awareness that you are doing so.

Irritable

PsyType: **4**
State: **Imbalanced in Courage**
Effect: **Negative**
Cause: Overdevelopment of the instinct to preserve the individual.

Definition: Quick excitability to annoyance, impatience or anger.

Isolation

PsyType: **9o**
State: **Imbalanced in Wisdom**
Effect: **Negative**
Cause: Undevelopment of the instinct to reason.

Definition: An individual socially withdrawn or removed from society.

Jealous

PsyType: **X**
Imbalance: **X**
Effect: **Negative**
Definition: Intolerant of rivalry or unfaithfulness; hostile attitude toward a rival or one believed to enjoy an advantage. Jealousy is desiring to see someone's advantage or blessing taken away. Manifesting this negative trait, you know no peace burning, as it were, in the fire of jealousy. Jealousy also destroys the value of your good works as a Tradition states: "Jealousy consumes positive traits as fire consumes wood."

Joker

PsyType: **4**
State: **Imbalanced in Courage**
Effect: **Negative**
Cause: Overdevelopment of the instinct to preserve the individual.

Definition: If jesting be employed in a measure of equilibrium, it is praiseworthy. To stand on the boundary of equilibrium is an extremely difficult thing to do. Most people aim at equilibrium but once under way, they overpass the boundary by such an encroachment that it becomes a reason for alarm. Latent anger is made apparent and a bitter, deep-seated ill-will takes firm root in people's hearts. Thus, jesting should not be done by someone who is not able to observe moderation. You sometimes begin jesting and do not know where to stop so you overstep the limit and endeavor to out-do your friends because of a sense of estrangement, the raising of a latent anger, and the sowing of a lasting hate, thus causing anger.

Joyful

PsyType: **6***
State: Balanced in Temperance
Effect: **Positive**
Definition: Experiencing or showing the emotion evoked by well-being, success, or good fortune or by the prospect of possessing what one desires.

Just, the (al-Adl)

PsyType: **9***
Effect: **Positive**
Quality: Cold
Prayer: Recite ya Adl on a

piece of bread on Thursday night and eat the bread and people should obey you.

King of Absolute Sovereignty
(Malik al-Mulk)
PsyType: 6*
Effect: Positive
Quality: Balanced in Hot/Cold
Prayer: Recite ya Malik al-Mulk frequently and one should gain esteem among people.

Knower, the (al-Alim)
PsyType: 9*
Effect: Positive
Quality: Balanced in Hot/Cold
Prayer: Repeat ya 'Alim 100 times after every prescribed prayer and God may give one spiritual 'unveiling' or intuition (*kashf*). If you want to know about hidden work, you should go down in prostration on Friday night and say ya Alim 100 times and sleep there. If you frequently recite ya Alim your heart may become illuminated. If you desire something, you should perform ablution, go to a forest, face the direction of prayer (*qiblah*), offer a two cycle prayer and then recite ya Alim 1000 times.

Languid, too
PsyType: 5
**State:Imbalanced in
      Temperance**
Effect: Negative
Cause: Underdevelopment in the instinct to preserve the species.
Definition: Sluggish in character or disposition.

Last, the (al-Akhir)
PsyType: 9*

Effect: Positive
Quality: Cold
Prayer: Those who recite ya Akhir frequently should lead a good life and have a good end at the time of death.

Lazy
PsyType: 5
**State: Imbalanced in
      Temperance**
Effect: Negative
Cause: Underdevelopment of the instinct to preserve the species.
Definition: Disinclined to activity or exertion; encouraging inactivity or insolence.

Liar
PsyType: 1
State: Imbalanced in Wisdom
Imbalance: C
Effect: Negative
Cause: Overdevelopment of the instinct to reason.
Definition: Marked by or containing falsehood.

Liberal
PsyType: 3*
State: Balanced in Courage
Effect: Positive
Definition: To be generous and openhanded.

Licentious (see Lust)
PsyType: 7
**State:Imbalanced in
      Temperance**
Effect: Negative
Cause: Overdevelopment of the instinct to preserve the species.
Definition: Lacking in moral restraint.

Life-Giver, the (al-Muhyi)

PsyType: 6*
Effect: Positive
Quality: Hot
Prayer: If you are weighed down with a heavy burden and repeat ya Muhyi seven times a day, you may have your burden removed.

Light, the (al-Nur)

PsyType: 9*
Effect: Positive
Quality: Hot
Prayer: Repeat ya Nur frequently and perhaps you will gain inner light. If you recite ya Nur 700 times on a Thursday night, you may receive inner light. If you recite Surah Nur seven times and ya Nur 1000 times you may gain light in your heart.

Living, the (al-Hayy)

PsyType: 9*
Effect: Positive
Quality: Balanced in Hot/Cold
Prayer: Recite ya Hayy frequently and you may gain a long life. If you are sick, you may be cured.

Lord of Majesty and Bounty
(Dhu 'l-Jalal wa 'l-Ikram)

PsyType: 9*
Effect: Positive
Quality: Hot
Prayer: Repeat ya Dhu 'l-Jalal wa 'l-Ikram frequently and you may develop esteem among people.

Loss of Self-Respect

PsyType: 7
State: Imbalanced in
        Temperance
Effect: Negative
Cause: Overdevelopment of the instinct to preserve the species.
Definition: Loss of proper respect for oneself as a human being; lack of regard for one's own standing or position.

Love of the World (see Love of Wealth and Riches)

PsyType: 7
State: Imbalanced in
        Temperance
Effect: Negative
Cause: Overdevelopment of the instinct to preserve the species.
Definition: Inordinate desire for things of this world. Quran: "*O believers, let not your wealth and your children distract you from remembrance of God. Those who do so, they are the losers*" (63:9). "*Decked out fair to mankind is love of lusts— women, children, stored-up heaps of gold and silver, horses of mark, cattle, and tillage. That is the enjoyment of the life of the world but God—with Him is the fairest resort*" (3:14). Tradition: "The love of wealth and position nourish hypocrisy just as plants are nourished by water." And, "How fair is rightly acquired wealth in the possession of an upright person."

Loving, the (al-Wadud)

PsyType: 3*
Effect: Positive
Quality: Balanced in Hot/Cold
Prayer: If there has been a quarrel between two people and one of the two repeats ya Wadud 1000 times over food and gives the food to the other to eat, the disagreement may be resolved.

Lust, Lack of Necessary

PsyType: 5
State: Imbalanced in

Temperance
Effect: Negative
Cause: Underdevelopment of
the instinct to preserve the species.
Definition: Lack of the neces-
sary desire to preserve the species.

Magnificent, the (al-Azim)
PsyType: 9*
Effect: Positive
Quality: Balanced in Hot/Cold
Prayer: Recite ya 'Azim fre-
quently and you may develop respect
among people.

Maintainer, the (al-Muqit)
PsyType: 3*
Effect: Positive
Quality: Hot
Prayer: If someone who is ill-
mannered, repeats ya Muqit several
times into a glass of water and drinks
it, the person may develop good manners.

Obstinate
PsyType: 5
State:Imbalanced in
   Temperance
Effect: Negative
Cause: Underdevelopment of
the instinct to preserve the species.
Definition: Perversely holding
to an opinion, purpose, or course of
action in spite of reason, arguments
or persuasion.

One, the (al-Ahad)
PsyType: 9*
Effect: Positive
Quality: Cold

Opener, the (al-Fattah)
PsyType: 3*
State: Balanced in Courage
Effect: Positive

Quality: Hot
Prayer: With hands on one's
chest, repeat ya Fattah 70 times after
teh dawn ritual prayer and rust should
go from your heart. It should open and
be given victory in the struggle to
morally heal.

Oppressive
PsyType: X
Imbalance: X
Effect: Negative
Definition: Unjust or cruel
exercise of authority or power; a sense
of being weighed down in body or
mind (depression).

Orderly
PsyType: 6*
State: Balanced in Temperance
Effect: Positive
Definition: Not marked by dis-
order.

Ostentatious (see Showing Off)
PsyType: 1
State: Imbalanced in Wisdom
Effect: Negative
Cause: Overdevelopment of the
instinct to reason.
Definition: Marked by preten-
tious display.

Overbearing
PsyType: 7
State: Imbalanced in
   Temperance
Effect: Negative
Cause: Overdevelopment of the
instinct to preserve the species.
Definition: Harshly and haugh-
tily arrogant.

Overconscious

PsyType: 1
State: Imbalanced in Wisdom
Effect: Negative
Cause: Overdevelopment of the instinct to reason.
Definition: Excess of the cognitive function.

Pardoner, the (al-Afu)

PsyType: 3*
State: Balanced in Courage
Effect: Positive
Quality: Hot
Prayer: Repeat frequently and one's wrongdoings should be forgiven.

Passive in Regard to Food, Sex, Earning a Living

PsyType: 5
State: Imbalanced in
　　　　Temperance
Effect: Negative
Cause: Underdevelopment of the instinct to preserve the species.
Definition: Passive and indifferent in regard to food, sex, or earning a living.

Patient, the (al-Sabur)

PsyType: 3*
State: Balanced in Courage
Effect: Positive
Quality: Hot
Prayer: Repeat thirty-three times and one should be rescued from troubles, difficulties or sorrow.

Patronizing

PsyType: 4
State: Imbalanced in Courage
Effect: Negative
Cause: Overdevelopment in the instinct to preserve the individual.
Definition: To adopt a superior air towards others.

Penetration of Idea

PsyType: 9*
State: Balanced in Wisdom
Effect: Positive
Definition: The ability to discern deeply and acutely.

Perceive Right from Wrong in all Voluntary Actions

PsyType: 9*
State: Balanced in Wisdom
Effect: Positive

Perplexed

PsyType: 1
State: Imbalanced in Wisdom
Effect: Negative
Cause: Overdevelopment of the instinct to reason.
Definition: To make unable to grasp something clearly or to think logically and decisively about something; to complicate.

Persist in Wrongdoing

PsyType: X
Imbalance: X
Effect: Negative

Pious

PsyType: 6*
State: Balanced
Imbalance: A
Effect: Positive

Postponer, the (al-Muakhkhir)

PsyType: 6*
State: Balanced in Temperance
Effect: Positive
Quality: Balanced in Hot/Cold
Prayer: Recite ya Mu'akhkhir 100 times in one's heart and only love

of God should remain. No other love can enter.

Powerful, the (al-Muqtadir)
PsyType: 6*
State:Balanced in Temperance
Effect: Positive
Quality: Cold
Prayer: Repeat ya Muqtadir frequently and one should become aware of the truth.

Praised, the (al-Hamid)
PsyType: 9*
State: Balanced in Wisdom
Effect: Positive
Prayer: Repeat ya Hamid frequently and one may be loved and praised.

Prayer, the Responder to
PsyType: 3*
State: Balanced in Courage
Effect: Positive
Quality: Hot
Prayer: Recite ya Mujib frequently and supplicate and one should continue to have faith.

Precise (see Correctness of Opinion)
PsyType: 9*
State: Balanced in Wisdom
Effect: Positive
Definition: Exactly defined or stated.

Preconscious
PsyType: 8
State: Imbalanced in Wisdom
Effect: Negative
Cause: Underdevelopment of the instinct to reason.
Definition: Not present in consciousness but capable of being recalled without encountering any inner resistance or repression.

Prejudiced
PsyType: 8
State: Imbalanced in Wisdom
Effect: Negative
Cause: Underdevelopment of the instinct to reason.
Definition: Preconceived judgment or opinion.

Preserver, the (al-Hafiz)
PsyType: 6*
State:Balanced in Temperance
Effect: Positive
Quality: Balanced in Hot/Cold
Prayer: Recite ya Hafiz sixteen times a day and one should be protected from calamities.

Presumptuous
PsyType: 4
State: Imbalanced in Courage
Effect: Negative
Cause: Overdevelopment of the instinct to preserve the individual.
Definition: To be presumptuous is to desire recompense in addition to thanks for a gift given.

Presumptiousness in devotional acts, according to Algazel, consists in a person's belief that by means of these he has acquired status with God and deserves special consideration from God in this life. You feel that undesirable events are less likely to happen to you than to a sinner. You expect God to accept your prayer more readily than a sinner's so that you are surprised when your own prayer is refused. You act if by your deeds you have done God a favor.

Prodigal

PsyType: 7
State: Imbalanced in
  Temperance
Effect: Negative
Cause: Overdevelopment of the
instinct to preserve the species.
  Definition: Recklessly extrava-
gant; characterized by wasteful expen-
diture.

Prevent the Negative
PsyType: 9*
State: Balanced in Wisdom
Effect: Positive
Definition: Guiding yourself and
others away from the development of
the negative.

Projection
PsyType: 9o
State: Imbalanced in Wisdom
Effect: Negative
Cause: Undevelopment in the
instinct to preserve the species.
  Definition: The attribution of
one's own ideas, feelings or attitudes
to other people or to objects; the
externalization of blame, guilt or
responsibility as a defense against
anxiety.

Promoter, the (al-Muqaddim)
PsyType: 6*
State: Balanced in Temperance
Effect: Positive
Quality: Cold
Prayer: Repeat ya Muqaddim
on the battlefield or when one is afraid
of being alone in frightening place
and no harm should come to one.

Protector, the (al-Mani)
PsyType: 6*
State:Balanced in Temperance
Effect: Positive

Quality: Hot
Prayer: Repeat ya Mani frequently and one should have a good
family life. Recite twenty times frequently and God should subside one's
anger.

Proud, the (al-Mutakabbir)
PsyType: 9*
State: Balanced in Wisdom
Effect: Positive
Quality: Hot
Prayer: Begin every act with ya
Mutakabbir and one may get one's
wish.

Provider, the (al-Razzaq)
PsyType: 3*
State: Balanced in Courage
Effect: Positive
Quality: Cold
Prayer: Standing and facing
the direction of prescribed prayer
repeat ya Razzaq 10 times to the four
directions while standing. Repeat frequently and you may not suffer poverty. Repeat 545 times frequently in the
direction of the qiblah and your sustenance should be met. Repeat 1000
times in seclusion and you may meet
Khidr (the inner guide). All of this is
conditional upon your earning your
sustenance (livelihood) in a permissi-
ble (*halal*) way

Quarrelsome
PsyType: 4
State: Imbalanced in Courage
Effect: Negative
Cause: Overdevelopment of the
instinct to preserve the individual.
  Definition: To complain. A
ground of dispute or complaint; alter-
cation.

Quest for Precious Things
> PsyType: 4
> State: Imbalanced in Courage
> Effect: Negative
> Cause: Overdevelopment of the
instinct to preserve the individual.
> Definition: Pursuing the collection of precious things becomes the cause for rivalry and argument. It also exposes one to the fear of loss or to the grief that is a necessary consequence of loss.

Quick-witted
> PsyType: 9*
> State: Balanced in Wisdom
> Effect: Positive
> Definition: Obtains when from much concern with conclusive premises.

Rationalization
> PsyType: 9o
> State: Imbalanced in Wisdom
> Effect: Negative
> Cause: Undevelopment of the instinct to reason.
> Definition: To attribute one's actions to rational and credible motives without analysis of them and especially unconscious motives; to provide plausible but untrue reasons for conduct.

Reaction Formation
> PsyType: 9o
> State: Imbalanced in Wisdom
> Effect: Negative
> Cause: Undevelopment of the instinct to reason.
> Definition: Response induced by vital resistance to another action.

Rebellious
> PsyType: X

> Imbalance: X
> Effect: Negative
> Definition: A form of arrogance. For the spiritual warrior, it is someone who rebels against God's Commands.
> Discussion: All mean outbreak against authority.

Recall
> PsyType: 9*
> State: Balanced in Wisdom
> Effect: Positive

Reckless
> PsyType: 4
> State: Imbalanced in Courage
> Effect: Negative
> Cause: Overdevelopment of the instinct to preserve the individual.
> Definition: Marked by lack of proper caution; careless of consequences. Reckless entrance into dangerous and deadly situations despite the warnings of reason.

Reckoner, the (al-Hasib)
> PsyType: 3*
> State: Balanced in Courage
> Effect: Positive
> Quality: Balanced in Hot/Cold
> Prayer: Repeat ya Hasib seventy times on Thursday during the day and night for 7 days and nights and the 71st time say, "God is my Reckoner." You should then be free of the fear of being robbed or being jealous of another or being harmed or wronged.

Remission in Important Affairs
> PsyType: 9o
> State: Imbalanced in Wisdom
> Effect: Negative

Cause: Undevelopment of the instinct to reason.

Definition: To lay aside a mood or disposition partly or wholly in dealing with important affairs; to desist from an activity, to let slacken.

Repentance, the Acceptor of

(al-Tawwab)

PsyType: 3*

State: Balanced in Courage

Effect: Positive

Quality: Hot

Prayer: Repeat ya Tawwab many times and one's repentance should be accepted.

Repression

PsyType: 9o

State: Imbalanced in Wisdom

Effect: Negative

Cause: Undevelopment of the instinct to reason.

Definition: A process by which unacceptable desires or impulses are excluded from consciousness and left to operate in the unconscious.

Resolute

PsyType: 6*

State:Balanced in Temperance

Effect: Positive

Definition: Marked by firm determination.

Resourceful, the (al-Wajid)

PsyType: 9*

State: Balanced in Wisdom

Effect: Positive

Quality: Balanced in Hot/Cold

Prayer: Repeat ya Wajid with every morsel of food one eats and one may become light.

Restorer, the (al-Muid)

PsyType: 6*

State: Balanced in Temperance

Effect: Positive

Quality: Balanced in Hot/Cold

Prayer: Repeat ya Mu'id seventy times for someone away from their family and they should return safely.

Resurrector, the (al-Ba'ith)

PsyType: 6*

State: Balanced in Temper ance

Effect: Positive

Quality: Balanced in Hot/Cold

Prayer: Frequently recite ya Ba'ith100 times and one should gain fear of God.

Retention

PsyType: 9*

State: Balanced in Wisdom

Effect: Positive

Retreating from Life (see Apathy)

PsyType: 5

State: Imbalanced in Temperance

Effect: Negative

Cause: Underdevelopment of the instinct to preserve the species.

Definition: Living apart from society.

Revengeful

PsyType: 4

State: Imbalanced in Courage

Effect: Negative

Cause: Overdevelopment of the instinct to preserve the individual.

Definition: To inflict injury in retaliation.

Rich, the (al-Ghani)

PsyType: 9*

State: Balanced in Wisdom
Effect: Positive
Quality: Hot
Prayer: Repeat ya Ghani frequently and one may become contented and not covetous.

Ridicule Others

PsyType: X
Imbalance: X
Effect: Negative
Definition: Making fun of others.

Discussion: This negative trait is usually caused by jealousy and enmity although it may also be rooted in greed, envy, or pride.

Sad (see Grieving)

PsyType: 60
State:Imbalanced in
       Temperance
Effect: Positive
Cause: Undevelopment of the instinct to preserve the species.
Definition: Affected with or expressive of grief or unhappiness.

Sarcastic (see Overconscious)

PsyType: 9*
State: Balanced in Wisdom
Effect: Positive
Definition: A sharp and often satirical utterance designed to cut or give pain.

Satanic Temptations

PsyType: 8
State: Imbalanced in Wisdom
Effect: Negative
Cause: Underdevelopment of the instinct to reason.
Definition:

Scorn, Being an Object of

PsyType: 4
State: Imbalanced in Courage
Imbalance: B
Effect: Negative
Cause: Overdevelopment of the instinct to preserve the individual.
Definition: Scorn is a trait of those who are given to impudence and nonsense. If you engage in scorn you apparently have no self-regard. You will appear to be very entertaining to others, provoking the laughter of the wealthy and the comfortably off. On the other hand, anyone marked by liberality and superiority will hold his own self and honor too dear to expose to even one impertinence from an impudent person.

Self-Abasing

PsyType: 2
State: Imbalance in Courage
Effect: Negative
Cause: Underdevelopment of the instinct to preserve the individual.
Definition: To lower self in rank, office, prestige or esteem.

Self-Alienating

PsyType: X
Imbalance: X
Effect: Negative
Definition: Withdrawing or separating of a person or his affections from an object of position of former attachment.

Self-Confidence, Lacking in

PsyType: 2
State: Imbalance in Courage
Effect: Negative
Cause: Underdevelopment of the instinct to preserve the individual.
Definition: Lacking confidence

in oneself and one's abilities and powers.

Self-Conscious (see Bashful)

PsyType: 2
State: Imbalance in Courage
Imbalance: B
Effect: Negative
Cause: Underdevelopment of the instinct to preserve the individual.
Definition: Uncomfortably conscious of self as an object of the observation of others.

Self-Debasing (see Self-Abasing)

PsyType: 2
State: Imbalance in Courage
Effect: Negative
Cause: Underdevelopment of the instinct to preserve the individual.
Definition: Self-inflicted or supposed loss of position, worth, value or dignity.

Self-Degrading (see Self-Abasing)

PsyType: 2
State: Imbalanced in Courage
Effect: Negative
Cause: Underdevelopment of the instinct to preserve the individual.
Definition: To drag down in moral or intellectual character; to bring to low esteem or into disrepute.

Self-Demeaning (see Self-Abasing)

PsyType: 2
State: Imbalanced in Courage
Effect: Negative
Cause: Underdevelopment of the instinct to preserve the individual.
Definition: To lower oneself below what it deserves.

Self-Esteem, Lack of

PsyType: 2
State: Imbalanced in Courage
Effect: Negative
Cause: Underdevelopment of the instinct to preserve the individual.
Definition: To fail to set a high value on self.

Self-Existing, the (al-Qayyum)

PsyType: 9*
State: Balanced in Wisdom
Effect: Positive
Quality: Hot
Prayer: Recite ya Qayyum at the time of the dawn prescribed prayer and people may keep you as a friend.

Self-Humiliating (see Self-Abasing)

PsyType: 2
State: Imbalanced in Courage
Effect: Negative
Cause: Underdevelopment of the instinct to preserve the individual.
Definition: To reduce oneself to a lower position in one's own eyes or others' eyes.

Self-Independent

PsyType: 6*
State: Balanced in Temperance
Effect: Positive
Definition: Being independent of others and indifferent to what is in their hands is opposite of greed and envy.

Self-Indulgent

PsyType: 7
State: Imbalanced in Temperance
Effect: Negative

Cause: Overdevelopment of the instinct to preserve the species.

Definition: Excessive or unrestrained gratification of one's own appetites, desires, or whims.

Self-Regard, Lack of (see Self-Esteem, Lack of)

PsyType: 2
State: Imbalanced in Courage
Effect: Negative
Cause: Underdevelopment of the instinct to preserve the individual.

Definition: Lack of self-respect or consideration of one's own interests.

Self-Restraining

PsyType: 6*
State: Balanced in Temperance
Effect: Positive
Definition: Temperant by restraining the self to moderation.

Self-Restraint, Excessive

PsyType: 5
State: Imbalanced in Temperance
Effect: Negative
Cause: Underdevelopment of the instinct to preserve the species.

Definition: Excessive restraining of the self from necessary pleasures.

Self-Sacrifice (see Altruistic)

PsyType: 3*
State: Balanced in Courage
Effect: Positive
Definition: Sacrificing oneself for others.

Self-Sufficient

PsyType: 9*
State: Balanced in Wisdom

Effect: Positive
Definition: Able to maintain oneself without outside aid.

Selfish

PsyType: 4
State: Balanced in Courage
Effect: Negative
Cause: Overdevelopment of the instinct to preserve the individual.

Definition: Concerned excessively or exclusively with oneself or one's will being without regard for others; arising from concern with one's own welfare or advantage in disregard of others.

Sexually Harass

PsyType: 7
State:Imbalanced in Temperance
Effect: Negative
Cause: Overdevelopment of the instinct to preserve the species.

Definition: To persistently annoy with sexual overtures.

Shameless

PsyType: 7
State:Imbalanced in Temperance
Effect: Negative
Cause: Overdevelopment of the instinct to preserve the species.

Definition: Insensible to disgrace.

Shaper of Unique Beauty, the
(al-Musawwir)

PsyType: 6*
State:Balanced in Temperance
Effect: Positive
Quality: Hot
Prayer: Recite ya Musawwir frequently and hard work should

become easy.

Showing Off

PsyType: 1
State: Balanced in Wisdom
Effect: Negative
Cause: Overdevelopment in the instinct to reason.
Definition: To display proudly; to seek to attract attention by conspicuous behavior.

Shrewd (see Cunning)

PsyType: 1
State: Imbalanced in Wisdom
Effect: Negative
Cause: Overdevelopment in the instinct to reason.
Definition: Stresses practical, hardheaded cleverness and judgment.

Sincere

PsyType: 9*
State: Balanced in Wisdom
Effect: Positive
Definition: Genuine in feeling with absence of hypocrisy or any falsifying embellishment or exaggeration.

Slanderer

PsyType: 1
State: Imbalanced in Wisdom
Effect: Negative
Cause: Overdevelopment of the instinct to reason.
Definition: The utterance of false charges or misrepresentations which defame and damage another's reputation; a false and defamatory oral statement about a person.

Slothful (see Lazy)

PsyType: 5
State: Imbalanced in Temperance

Effect: Positive
Cause: Underdevelopment of the instinct to preserve the species.
Definition: Spiritual apathy and inactivity.

Sluggishness of Appetite

PsyType: 5
State: Imbalanced in Temperance
Effect: Negative
Cause: Underdevelopment of the instinct to preserve the species.
Definition: Slow to respond to impulses of hunger.

Sly (see Cunning)

PsyType: 1
State: Imbalanced in Wisdom
Effect: Negative
Cause: Overdevelopment of the instinct to reason.
Definition: Human intellect so immersed in meticulous examination and analysis that it loses temperance.

Sovereign, the (al-Malik)

PsyType: 9*
State: Balanced in Wisdom
Effect: Positive
Quality: Cold
Prayer: Recite ya Malik frequently and one may be treated with respect by others.

Speed of Understanding

PsyType: 9*
State: Balanced in Wisdom
Effect: Positive

Spendthrift (see Prodigal)

PsyType: 7
State: Imbalanced in Temperance
Effect: Negative
Cause: Overdevelopment of the

instinct to preserve the species.

Definition: One who spends wastefully.

Spiritless

PsyType: 2
State: Imbalanced in Courage
Effect: Negative
Cause: Underdevelopment of the instinct to preserve the individual.

Definition: Lacking animation, cheerfulness, or courage. Lowering the self below what it deserves.

Squanderer (see Extravagant)

PsyType: 7
State:Imbalanced in
   Temperance
Effect: Negative
Cause: Overdevelopment of the instinct to preserve the species.

Definition: To spend extravagantly or foolishly.

Status Seeking

PsyType: 7
State: Imbalanced in
   Temperance
Effect: Negative
Cause: Overdevelopment of the instinct to preserve the species.

Definition: Seeking of position or rank in a hierarchy of prestige.

Stingy

PsyType: 5
State:Imbalanced in
   Temperance
Effect: Negative
Cause: Underdevelopment of instinct to preserve the species.

Definition: Sparing in giving or spending when reason dictates it is needed. A marked lack of generosity. Provided in meanly limited supply.

Stolid (see Impassive)

PsyType: 5
State: Imbalanced in Wisdom
Effect: Negative
Cause: Underdevelopment of the instinct to preserve the species.

Definition: That which arises from ill will and not from lack of natural disposition. Unemotional; impassive; having or expressing little or no sensibility.

Strong, the (al-Qawi)

PsyType: 9*
State: Balanced in Wisdom
Effect: Positive
Quality: Hot
Prayer: One who cannot defeat an enemy and repeats ya Qawi frequently with the intention of not being harmed should be freed of any harm by one's enemy.

Stubborn

PsyType: 5
State:Imbalanced in
   Temperance
Effect: Negative
Cause: Underdevelopment of the instinct to preserve the species.

Definition: Being unyielding and obstinate.

Subduer, the (al-Qahhar)

PsyType: 9*
State: Balanced in Wisdom
Effect: Positive
Quality: Balanced in Hot/Cold
Prayer: One who recites ya Qahhar 100 times between the obligatory and recommended dawn prayer should be able to overpower your enemy. If you repeat ya Qahhar frequently, you may conquer the desires

of the flesh—the passions—and your heart may become free of attractions to this world. You should gain inner peace and be freed from being wronged.

Superstitious (see Unconscious)

PsyType: 9o
State: Imbalanced in Wisdom
Effect: Negative
Cause: Undevelopment of the instinct to reason.
Definition: A belief or practice resulting from ignorance, fear of the unknown, trust in magic or chance, or a false conception of causation.

Teacher, the (al-Rashid)

PsyType: 6*
State: Balanced in Temperance
Effect: Positive
Quality: Balanced in Hot/Cold
Prayer: Repeat ya Rashid 1000 times between early evening prescribed prayer and the night prescribed prayer and one's troubles should clear up.

Temperance

PsyType: 6*
State: Balanced in Temperance
Effect: Positive

Timid (see Bashful)

PsyType: 2
State: Imbalanced in Courage
Effect: Negative
Cause: Underdevelopment of the instinct to preserve the individual.
Definition: Lacking in courage or self-confidence; boldness or determination.

Tolerant

PsyType: 9*
State: Balanced in Wisdom
Effect: Positive
Definition: Sympathy or indulgence for beliefs or practices differing from or conflicting with one's own.

Tranquil

PsyType: 6*
State: Balanced in Temperance
Effect: Positive
Definition: Free from disturbance or turmoil.

Troublemaker

PsyType: 4
State: Imbalanced in Courage
Effect: Negative
Cause: Overdevelopment of the instinct to preserve the individual.
Definition: Person who consciously or unconsciously causes trouble.

Trustee, the (al-Wakil)

PsyType: 3*
State: Balanced in Courage
Effect: Positive
Quality: Balanced in Hot/Cold
Prayer: If one is afraid of drowning, being burned in a fire or a similar danger, one should repeat ya Wakil from time to time to be under God's protection.

Truth, the (al-Haqq)

PsyType: 9*
State: Balanced in Wisdom
Effect: Positive
Prayer: One who recites ya Haqq should find something lost.

Truthful (see Truth)

PsyType: 9*

State: Balanced in Wisdom
Effect: Positive
Definition: Being in accord with fact or reality.

Unconsciousness
PsyType: 9o
State: Imbalanced in Wisdom
Effect: Negative
Cause: Undevelopment of the instinct to reason.
Definition: Not marked by conscious thought, sensation or feeling; not knowing or   perceiving; lack of self awareness.

Unemotional (see Impassiveness)
PsyType: 5
State: Imbalanced in Temperance
Effect: Negative
Cause: Underdevelopment of the instinct to preserve the species.
Definition: Lacking in emotions.

Unique, the (al-Wahid)
PsyType: 9*
State: Balanced in Wisdom
Effect: Positive
Quality: Balanced in Hot/Cold
Prayer: Recite ya Wahid 1000 times when one is alone and in a dark place and one should be freed of fear and delusions.

Unkind
PsyType: 4
State: Imbalanced in Courage
Effect: Negative
Cause: Overdevelopment of the instinct to preserve the individual.
Definition: Lacking in kindness or sympathy; harsh, cruel.

Unsociable
PsyType: 5
State: Imbalanced in Temperance
Effect: Negative
Cause: Underdevelopment of the instinct to preserve the species.
Definition: Lacking in a taste or desire for society or close association, having or showing a disinclination for social activity; solitary, reserved.

Usurer
PsyType: X
Imbalance: X
Effect: Negative
Definition: The lending of money with interest charged for its use.

Vain
PsyType: 4
State: Imbalanced in Courage
Effect: Negative
Cause: Overdevelopment of the instinct to preserve the individual.
Definition: Inflated pride in oneself or one's appearance; conceit.

Valor
PsyType: 3*
State: Balanced in Courage
Effect: Positive
Definition: Strength of mind or spirit that enables a person to encounter danger with firmness.

Vanity
PsyType: 4
State: Imbalanced in Courage
Effect: Negative
Definition: A false belief in yourself whereby your 'self' is held to belong to a rank which it does not

deserve. You deceive the self in what
you think of yourself. If Vanity
exists at the level of requiring medication, you need to become aware of the
self and the many negative traits
which blemish it. The self should be
made to realize that the positive traits
are divided among people—no one
can attain perfection without the positive traits of others. That is, your positive traits depend on others and not
just yourself.

Vast, the (al-Wasi)
PsyType: 9*
State: Balanced in Wisdom
Effect: Positive
Quality: Balanced in Hot/Cold
Prayer: Recite ya Wasi fre-
quently for those who have difficulty
earning a living and they should have
good earnings. God may give them
contentment and blessings.

Vigilant, the (al-Raqib)
PsyType: 3*
State: Balanced in Courage
Effect: Positive
Quality: Balanced in Hot/Cold
Prayer: Repeat ya Raqib seven
times for one's self, family and prop-
erty to be under God's protection.

Vindictive
PsyType: 4
State: Imbalanced in Courage
Effect: Negative
Cause: Overdevelopment of the
instinct to preserve the individual.
Definition: Disposed to seek
revenge.

Wasteful (see Prodigal)
PsyType: 7
State:Imbalanced in

Temperance
Effect: Negative
Cause: Overdevelopment of the
instinct to preserve the species.
Definition: To spend or use
blessings carelessly.

Whimsical
PsyType: 7
State:Imbalanced in
Temperance
Effect: Negative
Cause: Overdevelopment of the
instinct to reason.
Definition: A capricious or
eccentric and often sudden idea or
turn of the mind; fancy.

Wily (see Cunning)
PsyType: 1
State: Imbalanced in Wisdom
Effect: Negative
Cause: Overdevelopment of the
instinct to reason.

Wisdom
PsyType: 9*
Balance: Balanced in Wisdom
Effect: Positive
Definition: A wise attitude or
course of action.

Wise, the (al-Hakim)
PsyType: 9*
State: Balanced in Wisdom
Effect: Positive
Quality: Balanced in Hot/Cold
Prayer: Recite frequently and
you should be able to overcome diffi-
culties in your work.

Witness, the (al-Shahid)
PsyType: 3*
State: Balanced in Courage
Effect: Positive
Quality: Hot

Prayer: Repeat ya Shahid twenty-one times with one's hand on a rebellious child's forehead and the child may become obedient.

Witty

PsyType: 6*

State:Balanced in Temperance

Effect: Positive

Definition: Cleverness and quickness of mind.

Zeal

PsyType: 3*

State: Balanced in Courage

Effect: Positive

Definition: Allow no indifference in preserving the integrity of religion and honor but to hold it right in such accounts; to push exertion to its furtherest limits.

Notes

Part I: Morality, the Law and the Way

1. See Ardalan and Bakhtiar, *The Sense of Unity: The Sufi Tradition in Persian Architecture* for a full explanation of how the Way is expressed in architecture.

Part II: Spiritual Chivalry
Chapter 1: The Goal

1. Kāshānī, *Tuḥfat al-ikhwan*, pp. 4-5. See S. Murata's *The Tao of Islam*, pp. 267-269. 'Abd al-Razzāq Kāshānī (d. 1335 AD) is one of the best known commentators on Ibn al-'Arabī's *Fuṣūs al-ḥikam* (*Bezels of Wisdom*).

2. Muḥāsibī, *Kitāb al-ri'āya*, fol. 100a. Ḥārith b. Asad al-Muḥāsibī (b. 781 AD) has long been recognized as the real master of early Islamic mysticism. "A study of al-Muḥāsibī's writings proves conclusively that he was the precursor of al-Ghazāli in giving to Sufi mysticism an assured place in orthodox Islam, and that al-Muḥāsibī's teaching formed the basis of much of the teaching of the greatest of the Muslim mystics, both Arab and Persian, who succeeded him, and especially of those who, in their turn, influenced the Christian scholastics.' See M. Smith, *An Early Mystic of Baghdad*, London: Sheldon Press, 1977.

3. See S. H. Nasr. Spiritual Chivalry. In *Islamic Spirituality:*

Manifestations, p. 315, n. 6.

4. Muḥāsibī, *Risālat ādāb al-nufūs*, fol. 63 b.

5. *Ibid.*

6. A Divine Tradition (*ḥadīth qudsī*) is one in which the Divinity spoke to the Messenger in the first person.

7. Muḥāsibī, *Kitāb al-ri'āya,*, fol. 12a.

8. Nasr, *Man and Nature*, p. 96.

Chapter 2: The Heart

1. Chittick, *The Sufi Path of Knowledge*, p. 106.

2. *Ibid.*, p. 107.

3. Muḥāsibī, *Kitāb al-ri'āya*, fol. 110a.

4. Chittick, *The Sufi Path of Knowledge*, p. 107.

5. *Ibid.*

6. *Ibid.*

7. *Ibid.*

8. Muḥāsibī, *Maḥāsabat al-nufūs,* fol. 5.

9. *Ibid.*

10. Hujwīrī, *Kashf al-maḥjūb*, p. 277. 'Alī ibn 'Uthmān Hujwīrī (d. 1072 AD) is author of one of the earliest Persian manuals of Sufi teaching, the *Kashf al-maḥjūb*.

11. Suhrāwardī, *Awārif al-ma'ārif*. Cairo: 1272. Shihāb al-Din Abū Hafṣ Suhrāwardī is the nephew of the founder of the Suhrawardī Sufi order. His *'Awārif al-ma'ārif* (Gifts of Mystic Knowledge) is considered to be a classic of Sufi practical and ethical teachings.

12. Izutsu, *Ethico-Religious*

Concepts in the Quran, p. 125.

13. Chittick, *The Sufi Path of Knowledge,* p. 65.

14. Anṣārī, *Ṣad maydān,* pp. 362-63. Khwāja 'Abdallāh Anṣārī (d. 1088) is a well known author of intimate prayers (*munājāt*) as well as an influential writer on the spiritual stations.

15. Anṣārī, *Manāzil al-sā'irin,* pp. 47-48.

16. Suhrawardī, p. 25. Abū al-Najīb Suhrawardī (d. 1097 AD) is the founder of the Suhrawardī Sufi order. He is considered to be an example of a typical representative of orthodox Sufism "combining legal and theological scholarship with mystical devotion, retirement from the world (as a temporary stage), and constant dedication to teaching and guiding the many." See *A Sufi Rule for Novices,* p. v.

CHAPTER 3: SPIRITUAL MODELS

1. Ibn al-'Arabī, *Tafsīr al-qur'ān al-karīm.,* Vol. 1, pp. 766 ff. Muḥyī al-Din Ibn al-'Arabī (d. 1240 AD) is known as the "Greatest Master," of Islamic mysticism. He brought together all the Islamic sciences in a synthesis that has influenced the Islamic world since his time. This work is said to have been done by his student, Kāshānī, in his name.

2. *Ibid.*

CHAPTER 4: SPIRITUAL STAGES

1.Ibn al-'Arabī, *Futūḥat,* II 588. 6.

In Murata, *The Tao of Islam,* p. 268.

2. *Ibid.*

3. Lane, *Lexicon* under *mr'*.

4. See the Quran, 17:1.

5. See the Quran, 12:24.

6. See the Quran, 38:17.

7. See the Quran, 38:41.

8. See the Quran, 37:122.

9. See the Quran, 37:133.

10. See the Quran, 17:65.

11. Anṣārī, *Ṣad maydān,* pp. 253-54.

12. Muḥāsībī, *Risālat ādāb al-nufūs,* fol. 72 b.

13. *Ibid.*

14. Anṣārī, *Ṣad maydān,* pp. 362-63.

15. Muḥāsībī, *Risālat ādāb al-nufūs,* fol. 58 b.

16. *Ibid.*

17. See 17:35.

18. Muḥāsībī, *Risālat ādāb al-nufūs,* fol. 47b.

19. *Ibid.*

20. *Ibid.*

21. *Ibid.*

22. Hujwīrī, *Kashf al-maḥjūb,* p. 249.

23. Muḥāsībī, *Risālat ādāb al-nufūs,* fol. 48 b.

24. Qushayrī, *Risāla,* pp. 472-73.

25. Muḥāsībī, *Risālat ādāb al-nufūs,* fol. 84 b.

26. *Ibid.*

27. Qushayrī, *Risāla,* pp. 472-73. Abu'l Qāsim al-Qushayrī (d. 1072) is author of one of the most important early works on Sufi biography and teachings.

28. Suhrawardī, *Rule for Sufi*

Novices.
29. *Ibid.*
30. Muḥāsibī, *Riṣālat ādāb al-nufūs*, fol. 44 b.
31. Nurbakhsh, Javad. The Nimatullāhī. In Nasr (Ed.) *Islamic Spirituality: Manifestations*, p. 159.

CHAPTER 5:
SPIRITUAL PRACTICES
1. Algazel. *Kīmiyā-yi sa'ādat*, pp. 13-16.
2. *Ibid.*

PART III: CAUSES OF MORAL IMBALANCES
CHAPTER 1: INTRODUCTION
1. Shah Walīullāh, *Altāf al-quds*, p. 36. Shah Waliullāh (b. 1702) was a Sufi of the highest rank.
2. *Ibid.*

CHAPTER 2:
PASSIONS VS. REASON
1. Muḥāsibī, *Kitāb al-ri'āya*, fol. 52b.
2. *Ibid.*
3. *Ibid.*
4. *Ibid.*
5. *Ibid.*
6. *Ibid.*
7. Shāh Walīullāh, *Altāf al-quds*, p. 40.

CHAPTER 3: IGNORANCE (JAHL) OF REALITY
1. See the Quran, 96:6.
2. See the Quran, 6:116.
3. Seethe Quran, 5:52.
4. See the Quran, 16:3-18.

5. See the Quran, 16:83.
6. See the Quran, 41:5.
7. See the Quran, 2:7.
8. See the Quran, 83:14.
9. See the Quran, 50:36.
10. See the Quran, 6:25.
11. Seethe Quran, 9:8.
12. Shāh Walīullāh, *SAltāf al-quds*, p. 46.
13. See the Quran, 13:14.
14. See the Quran, 24:40.
15. See the Quran, 31:11.
16. See the Quran, 40:45.
17. See the Quran, 42:27.
18. See the Quran, 7:143-44.
19. See the Quran, 42:42.
20. See the Quran, 25:21.
21. See the Quran, 40:4
22. See the Quran, 2:105.
23. See the Quran, 28:58.

PART IV: OBSERVING MORAL BALANCE IN NATURE
CHAPTER 1: LEARNING TO READ THE SIGNS
1. Ardalan and Bakhtiar, *The Sense of Unity*, p. 21.
2. *Ibid.* p. 25.
3. Nasr, S. H. Foreword to *Islamic Patterns*, p. 3.
4. Nicomachus, *Introduction to Arithmetic*, pp. 1813-14.
5. Haydar Amulī, *Ta'wīlāt*, fol. 669.
6. Schuon, *Gnosis: Divine Wisdom*, p. 113, n. 1.
7. Birūnī, *Alberuni's India*, pp. 294-295.

CHAPTER 2: MICROCOSM-

MACROCOSM

1. Ikhwān al-Ṣafā, *Rasā'il*, II, 20. In Nasr, *Introduction to Islamic Cosmological Doctrines*, p. 68. The Ikhwān lived in the 10th century AD. Known as the Brethren of Purity, they rewrote Neoplatonic and Pythagorean natural philosophy and metaphysics in Islamic terms in a series of about fifty treatises.

2. Nicholson, *Rumi, Mystic and Poet*, p. 124.

3. Smith, *al-Ghazzali, the Mystic*, p. 111.

4. Shabistari, *Gulsan-i-rāz*. In Nasr, *Science and Civilization in Islam*, pp. 15-16.

5. Bernnoulli, Rudolf. *Spiritual Development in Alchemy*. Eranos.

6. *Ibid.*

7. *Ibid.*

8. *Ibid.*

9. *Ibid.*

10. Corbin, *Temple and Contemplation*, p. 29.

11. Nasr, *Introduction to Islamic Cosmological Doctrines*, p. 165.

12. Critchlow, *Islamic Patterns*, p. 58.

13. *Ibid.*, p. 9.

14. *Ibid.*

15. Ardalan and Bakhtiar, *The Sense of Unity*, p. 27.

16. *Ibid.*, p. 48.

17. *Ibid.*, p. 49.

18. Ikhwan. In Nasr, *Introduction to Islamic Cosmological Doctrines*, p. 50.

19. Corbin, *Temple and Contemplation*, p. 68.

20. Critchlow, *Islamic Patterns*, pp. 9.

21. *Ibid.*

22. Ardalan and Bakhtiar, *The Sense of Unity*, p. 29.

23. Smith, *al-Ghazzali, the Mystic*, pp. 111-12.

24. Corbin, *Temple and Contemplation*, p. 230.

25. *Ibid.*

26. Iamblichius. *Theology of Arithmetic*, p. 105-6.

27. See the Quran, 7:107.

28. See the Quran, 7:108.

29. See the Quran, 7:130.

30. See the Quran, 7:130.

31. See the Quran, 7:133.

32. Ibn al-'Arabī, *Tafsīr al-quran al-karīm*.

33. Critchlow, *Islamic Patterns*, pp. 58.

34. Corbin, *Temple and Contemplation*, pp. 75.

35. Burckhardt, *Mystical Astrology*, pp. 26.

36. Critchlow, *Islamic Patterns*, p. 60.

37. Corbin, *Temple and Contemplation*, p. 78.

38. *Ibid.* It is interesting to note in this regard that Ibn al-'Arabī says the world began in the Sign of Libra, that the Messenger Muhammad was born in the Sign of Libra and that the world will end in the Sign of Libra.

39. Critchlow, *Islamic Patterns*, p. 154.

40. Burckhardt, *Mystical Astrology*, p. 41.

41. Corbin, *Temple and*

Contemplation, pp. 91.

42. Critchlow, *Islamic Patterns*, pp. 43, 46.

43. The author would like to acknowledge her gratitude to Keith Critchlow who was the first to her knowledge to have understood the importance of the coordination of Saturn and Jupiter for the traditional concepts of numbers and geometry. but he did not make the connection to it as the macrocosmic correspondence of the microcosmic Sign of the Presence of God, the origin of the Enneagram which this author has done based on traditional sources.

44. Critchlow, *Islamic Patterns*, p. 154.

45. Rumi, *Fihī mā fīhī*, p. 283.

46. Attar, *Ilāhināmah*, p. 328.

PART V: ATTAINING MORAL BALANCE THROUGH NURTURE
CHAPTER 1: INTRODUCTION

1. Algazel, *Ihyā Ulūm al-Din*, p. 127.

2. *Ibid.*

CHAPTER 2: COGNITIVE TECHNIQUES

1. See the Quran, 4:157.
2. See the Quran, 10:36.
3. See the Quran, 6:98.
4. See the Quran, 10:24.
5. See the Quran, 3:191.
6. See the Quran, 12:185.
7. Ibn Miskawayh, *Tahdhib*, p. 30. For a brief biography see *God's Will Be Done: Traditional Psychoethics and Personality*

Paradigm.

8. *Ibid.*
9. *Ibid.*
10. *Ibid.*
11. *Ibid.*
12. Makki, *Qut*, I 114, p. 18. Abū ˘alib al-Makkī (d. 996 AD) has written one of the first comprehensive manuals of Sufi practical and psychological teachings.

CHAPTER 3: BEHAVIORAL TECHNIQUES

1. See the Quran, 2:213.
2. See the Quran, 4:1.
3. See the Quran, 49:10.
4. See the Quran, 48:29.
5. See the Quran, 2:224.
6. See the Quran, 4:114.
7. See the Quran, 5:3.
8. Ibn Miskawayh, *Tahdhib*, p. 45.
9. *Ibid.*
10. *Ibid.*
11. *Ibid.*
12. Abu Dawud, *Adab*, 49; Tirmidhi, *Birr*, 18.
13. Ibn Miskawayh, *Tahdhib*, p. 48.

CHAPTER 4: AFFECTIVE TECHNIQUES

1. Rumi, Mathnawi IV, 276.
2. Ibn Miskawayh, *Tahdhib*, p. 72.

CHAPTER 5: MIXED TECHNIQUES

1. Ibn Miskawayh, *Tahdhib*, p. 75.

**Part VI: Attaining Moral
Balance Through the Sign
of the Presence of God
Chapter 1: The Healing
Work**

1. Tūsī, *Akhlaq*, p. 175.
2. *Ibid.*
3. *Ibid.*
4. *Ibid.*
5. *Ibid.*
6. Makkī, *Qut*, p. 20.
7. Tūsī, *Akhlaq*, p. 182.
8. *Ibid.*
9. *Ibid.*
10. *Ibid.*

**Chapter 3: Avoidance of
Harm/Pain Imbalances**

1. See the Quran, 8:46.
2. See the Quran, 3:146.
3. See the Quran, 47:35.
4. See the Quran, 4:77.
5. See the Quran, 3:175.

BIBLIOGRAPHY

al-Birūnī, *Al-Beruni's India: An Account of the Religion,
Philosophy, Literature, Geography, Chronology, Astronomy, Custom,
Laws and Astrology of India.* 2 vols. Translated by E. C. Sachau.
Longon: Kegan Paul, Trench, Trubner & Co., 1910.

al-Birūnī, *Elements of Astrology.* Translated by R. Ramsey Wright.
London, 1934.

Algazel. *Kīmiyā-yi sā'dat.* Edited by H. Khajiwjam. Tehran: Jībī, 1975.

Anṣārī, Khwāja. *Ṣad maydān.* Edited by R. Farhādī. In *Manāzil al-sā'rīn.*
Kabul: Bayhaqī, 1976.

Ardalan, N. and Bakhtiar, L. *The Sense of Unity: The Sufi Tradition in
Persian Architecture.* Chicago: University of Chicago Press, 1973.

Aṭṭār, Farīd al-Dīn. *Illāhīnāma.* Tehran, 1967.

Bakhtiar, Laleh. *God's Will Be Done: Traditional Psychoethics and
Personality Paradigm.* Vol. 1. Chicago: The Institute of Traditional
Psychoethics and Personality Paradigm, 1993.

Bakhtiar, Laleh. *SUFI Expressions of the Mystic Quest.* London: Thames
and Hudson, 1976.

Bernnoulli, Rudolf. Spiritual Development in Alchemy. Eranos.

Burckhardt, Titus. *Mystical Astrology.* London: Beshara Publications, 1967.

Chittick, William. *The Sufi Path of Knowledge.* NY: SUNY Press, 1989.

Corbin, Henri. *Temple and Contemplation.* London: KPI, 1986.

Hand, Robert. *World Ephemeris for the 20th Century.* Boston, MA:
Para Research, 1983.

Hujwīrī, Jullabī, al-. *Kashf al-maḥjūb.* Translated by R. A. Nicholson,
London: 1911.

Iamblichus. *The Theology of Arithmetic.* Translated by Robin Waterfield.
Grand Rapids, MI: Phanes Press, 1988.

Ibn al-'Arabī. *Tafsīr al-qur'ān al-karīm.* 2 vols. Beirut: 1968.

Izutsu, Toshihiko. *Ethico-Religious Concepts in the Quran.* Montreal,
Canada: McGill University Press, 1966.

Kāshānī, 'Abd al-Razzāq. *Tuḥfat al-ikhwān fī khaṣa'iṣ al-fityān.* In
Rasa'il-i jawān mardān. Edited by M. Ṣarrāf. Tehran: Institut Franco-
Iranien, 1973.

Lane, E. W. *Arabic-English Lexicon.* Cambridge, England: Islamic Texts
Society, 1984.

Makki, Abū Ṭālib. *Qūt al-qulūb.* Cairo: Muṣṭāfā al-Bābī al-Ḥalābī, 1961.

Miskāwayh, Ibn. *Tahdhīb al-akhlāq.* Translated by Constantine
Zurayk. Beirut, American University of Beirut, 1968.

Muḥāsībī, Ḥārith b. Asad. *Muḥāsabal al-nufūs.* MS, Cairo, Tas.
Sh. 3.

Muḥāsibī, Ḥārith b. Asad. *Kitāb al-ri'āya*. MS. Oxford, Hunt. 611.

Muḥāsibī, Ḥārith b. Asad. *Risālat ādāb al-nufūs*. MS. Istanbul, Jārallāh.

Murata, Sachiko. *The Tao of Islam: A Sourcebook for Gender Relationships in Islamic Thought*. NY: SUNY Press, 1992.

Nasr, S. H. *A Young Muslim's Guide to the Modern World*. Chicago: KAZI Publications, Inc. 1993.

Nasr, S. H. *Introduction to Islamic Cosmological Doctrines*. NY: SUNY, 1993.

Nasr. S. H. (Ed.) *Islamic Spirituality: Manifestations*. NY: Crossroads, 1991.

Nasr, S. H. *Man and Nature*. Kuala Lumpur, Malaysia: Foundation for Traditional Studies, 1976.

Nasr, S. H. *Science and Civilization in Islam*. Cambridge, England. Islamic Texts Society, 1987.

Nicholson, R. *Rumi, Poet and Mystic*. London: George Allen and Unwin, 1964.

Nicomachus, Introduction to Arithmetic. In *Encyclopedia Britannica*. Chicago: Encyclopedia Britannica, 1953.

Qushayrī, Abu'l Qāsim, al-. *al-Risāla*. Edited by 'Abd al-Ḥalīm Maḥmūd and Maḥmūd ibn al-Sharif. Cairo: Dār al-Kutub al-Ḥadītha, 1972.

Schuon, Fritjof. *Gnosis, Divine Wisdom*. Translated by G. E. H. Palmer. NY: Sophia Perennis et Universalis, 1993.

Shah, Waliullāh, Aḥmad. *Altāf al-quds fī ma'rifat latāif nafs*. Dehli, India: Dehlevi Publishers, 1976.

Smith, Margaret. *An Early Mystic of Baghdad*. London: Sheldon Press, 1977.

Smith, Margaret. *Al-Ghazzali, the Mystic*. London: Luzac and Co., 1944.

Suhrawardī, Abū al-Najīb. *Kitāb Adāb al-Murīdīn (A Sufi Rule for Novices)*. Cambridge, MA: Harvard University Press, 1975.

Rūmī, Jalāl al-Din. *Mathnawī*. Translated by R. A. Nicholson. 8 vols. London: E. J. Gibb, 1968.

Tūsī, N. *Akhlaq al-Nasīrī*. Translated by G. Wickens. London: George Allen & Unwin, 1964.

Index